DATE DUE

DEMCO, INC. 38-2931

Milieu Therapy: Significant Issues and Innovative Applications

Milieu Therapy: Significant Issues and Innovative Applications

Jerome M. Goldsmith, EdD
Jacquelyn Sanders, PhD
Editors

The Haworth Press, Inc.
New York • London • Norwood (Australia)

1697626   3-11-94

Milieu Therapy: Significant Issues and Innovative Applications has also been published as *Residential Treatment for Children & Youth*, Volume 10, Number 3 1993.

The Haworth Press, Inc., 10 Alice Street, Binghamton, NY 13904-1580 USA

Library of Congress Cataloging-in-Publication Data

Milieu therapy : significant issues and innovative applications / Jerome M. Goldsmith, Jacquelyn Sanders, editors.
      p. cm.
      "Has also been published as Residential treatment for children & youth, volume 10, number 3, 1993"–T.p. verso.
      Includes bibliographical references.
      ISBN 1-56024-409-7 (acid-free paper)
      1. Milieu therapy. 2. Child psychotherapy–Residential treatment. 3. Bettelheim, Bruno. 4. Universities and colleges–Psychological aspects. 5. College students–Mental health. I. Goldsmith, Jerome M. II. Sanders, Jacquelyn Seevak.
RJ505.M54M55 1993
618.92′89144–dc20
                                           93-15448
                                              CIP

Milieu Therapy: Significant Issues and Innovative Applications

CONTENTS

ABOUT THE EDITORS

Jerome M. Goldsmith, EdD, has had a distinguished career in residential treatment services for children, starting as Group Therapist in adolescent programs of the Jewish Board of Guardians, becoming Director of the Hawthorne Cedar-Knolls School for Severely Disturbed Adolescent Boys and Girls, and retiring in 1990 as Executive Vice-President of the JBG. He has had many teaching posts, including Adjunct professor at the New York University School of Social Work, many professional appointments, many honors, many organizational positions including President of the American Association of Children's Residential Centers, and has published widely. He recently served as a member of Mayor Dinkin's Commission for the Homeless.

Jacquelyn Sanders, PhD, was Director of the Sonia Shankman Orthogenic School of the University of Chicago between 1972 and 1992. Earlier she had worked with Bruno Bettelheim at the Orthogenic School as Counselor and Assistant Principal from 1952 to 1965. She is a licensed psychologist and has appointments at the University of Chicago as Senior Lecturer in the Department of Education and as Clinical Associate Professor in the Department of Psychiatry. She is currently president of the American Association of Children's Residential Treatment Centers.

ABOUT THE CONTRIBUTORS

D. Patrick Zimmerman, PsyD, is Coordinator of Research at the Sonia Shankman Orthogenic School and Lecturer in the Department of Psychiatry at the University of Chicago. He is also a member of the Senior Associate Faculty at the Illinois School for Professional Psychology and a candidate at the Chicago Center for Psychoanalysis. He is the founder of the Southern School, an alternative day school for disturbed inner city adolescents, and has published in a variety of professional journals.

Joseph Noshpitz is Psychiatrist-in-Chief, Chesapeake Youth Center, Cambridge, MD, and Clinical Professor of Psychiatry and Behavioral Science, George Washington University, Washington, DC. He is a Past President of the American Academy of Child and Adolescent Psychiatry and of the American Association of Children's Residential Centers. A practicing child psychiatrist and psychoanalyst, he has done extensive research in the areas of residential treatment, childhood gender development, anorexia, and narcissistic character disorder. His other publications include Stressors and Adjustment Disorders (Wiley, 1989) and Basic Handbook of Child Psychiatry, Volumes I-V, of which he is Editor-in-Chief.

Bertram J. Cohler is William Rainey Harper Professor in the College and Professor in the Departments of Psychology (The Committee on Human Development), Psychiatry, and Education at the University of Chicago. He is Resident Head, Linn House, Burton-Judson Courts in the University of Chicago Residence System.

Susan E. Taber is a Doctoral Student in The Committee on Human Development at the University of Chicago and Resident Head at Blackstone Hall in the University of Chicago Residence System.

Bettelheim Tribute

In the 1950's the American Association of Children's Residential Centers had among its ardent and thoughtful founders several men and women who gathered once each year at the University of Chicago campus. They would present ideas, practices and theories relevant to their work with disturbed children in residence. Among that group and one of the original founders of the Association was Bruno Bettelheim.

After Bruno Bettelheim's death, there was a flood of accounts that both extolled and discredited his contributions. This edition of the Association's publication plays no part in that disquisition.

We have invited authors to present papers illuminating our continuing efforts to further our understanding of the caring process and its impact upon the healing and repair measures for disturbed children.

Bruno Bettelheim is paid tribute by these presentations. For, no matter what the assessment history will accord to Bruno Bettelheim, his activities, his writings, his articulation of the importance of the hour by hour and day by day management of the child's daily living experiences will have forever changed our perception of the treatment of children. Further, his attribution of a critical therapeutic role to the caretaker has profoundly influenced treatment as well as recruitment and training of the child care counselor/caretaker for all time.

With respect and admiration for his contribution to the work of healing troubled children, we dedicate this publication to the memory of Bruno Bettelheim.

Jerome M. Goldsmith, EdD

1

The Clinical Thought
of Bruno Bettelheim:
A Critical Historical Review

D. Patrick Zimmerman, PsyD

SUMMARY. The present study surveys a selected number of Bruno Bettelheim's political and clinical articles. It begins with a brief presentation of biographical notes, derived from various published interviews with Dr. Bettelheim and from the articles chosen for review. Second, it presents a discussion of his political writings, which in this study include his observations about the psychological effects of the Nazi concentration camps, his research on ethnic prejudice, and his arguments against the Vietnam war protesters. Third, it discusses various clinical articles, focusing on his commentaries on milieu therapy and early case studies of childhood schizophrenia and autism. The paper concludes with a consideration of some of Bettelheim's personal attitudes during his final years.

INTRODUCTION

Many of Bruno Bettelheim's contributions to the conceptual refinements of milieu treatment remain with us even today as an

Earlier versions of this paper were presented at the 34th Annual Meeting of the American Association of Children's Residential Centers in St. Petersburg, Florida, October 11, 1990 and at the 99th Annual Convention of the American Psychological Association in San Francisco, California, August 20, 1991. This study was published previously in *Psychoanalysis and Contemporary Thought*, 14 (4), 1991, and is reprinted with permission from the publishers.

The author expresses gratitude to Aaron A. Hilkevitch, MD (Chicago), and Jacquelyn Seevak Sanders, PhD, Director of the Sonia Shankman Orthogenic School.

influential part of both the residential and inpatient care of children and adolescents in the United States and abroad. In an attempt to distill and clarify certain areas of Dr. Bettelheim's clinical legacy, especially in light of the intense controversies that have emerged about him after his death, the present study surveys a selected number of Bruno Bettelheim's political and clinical articles. It begins with a brief presentation of biographical notes, derived from various published interviews with Dr. Bettelheim and from the articles chosen for review. Second, it presents a critical reconstruction and evaluation of both the historical development and theoretical foundations of Bettelheim's writings in a number of areas, including: the psychological effects of the Nazi concentration camp experiences, ethnic prejudice, the Vietnam War protest, milieu therapy, childhood schizophrenia and autism, and his understanding of certain basic psychoanalytic concepts. An attempt is made to present a picture of certain connections between Bettelheim's own experiences and personality, and his political and clinical writings, which seemed to emerge in the course of this review. In addition, the study suggests how those connections may have both influenced and limited Bettelheim's understanding of certain important clinical concepts. Finally, the paper speculates about some of Bettelheim's personal attitudes during his final years, as they are suggested in his later works.

BIOGRAPHICAL NOTES

In 1987, I began collecting the wide–ranging published papers of Dr. Bettelheim with the perhaps overly ambitious aim of writing a comprehensive historical account of the development of his ideas and contributions with regard to the fields of psychology, education, and the therapeutic treatment of emotionally disturbed children. Even before Dr. Bettelheim's suicide and the subsequent controversies about him, I found myself experiencing reluctance about undertaking such a study (which would unavoidably involve an evaluation of aspects of his personality, related biographical data, and his historical importance).

In Kohut's (1976) reflections on Freud's self-analysis, he pointed out that "it is always hard to achieve an objective evaluation of a great man, whether the evaluation be by the average biographer, the historian, or the depth psychologist" (p. 172). This is so, according to Kohut, since the great man is likely to become a transference figure for the investigator (usually, a father figure), and the childhood ambivalences of the investigator may well intrude to distort or falsify the results. In Kohut's view, we are prone to establish an idealizing transference toward him, or to defend ourselves against it by a process of reaction formation. Further, the very choice of the biographical subject can be too strongly determined by the researcher's own identification tendencies. Finally, Kohut observed, the long study and preoccupation with the life of the person being investigated is prone to reinforce the bonds of identification even further.

That Bettelheim was sensitive to the immense difficulties in such an undertaking is clear from the beginning of the introduction to his final published work, *Freud's Vienna and Other Essays*, where he began by reminding the reader of Freud's cautions about biographical studies: "As a Freudian, I believe what Freud said about biographies applies even more to autobiographies, namely that the person who undertakes such a task binds himself to lying, to concealment, to flummery' " (Bettelheim, 1990, p. ix). Nevertheless, Bettelheim gave us this final book of essays as an autobiographical statement, though one in the form of a collection of essays, the selection and arrangement of which was intended to convey to the discerning reader ideas concerning the major influences in his life.

Bettelheim's comments in his final book about Ernest Jones's last years suggest an awareness that the end of his own life was approaching and that with diminished capacities he was working against time. Further, just as Bettelheim concluded that the importance of Freud and of correctly understanding him took precedence over a more sentimental appraisal of Jones's biography, so a sometimes critical review of Bettelheim might be justified, on the basis that he himself was, in a sense, not just another man, but rather one who was at least popularly viewed as one of the major influences on modern thought about children and the treatment of disturbed children.

Bruno Bettelheim was born in 1903 to an upper-middleclass Jewish family in Vienna. He remembered fondly the life experiences of both his grandfathers, as passed on to him as part of his family's oral history. His maternal grandfather was said to have been sent out alone into the world soon after his thirteenth birthday, with only one good suit of clothing and a silver piece worth about two and a half dollars. According to Bettelheim, in order to protect his only pair of shoes, the boy walked barefoot the hundred miles from his village to Vienna, where over the years he managed to make a great fortune. His paternal grandfather was raised from infancy in a Jewish orphanage. After it was discovered that he was very bright, he was being educated to become a rabbi when he was chosen by Baron Rothschild of Vienna to become the tutor of his sons. Many years later, when his charges had become leaders of the Rothschild bank, they put him in charge of many of its operations. Both tales left Bettelheim with the feeling that "nowhere else but in Vienna, or in a fairy-tale place, could a cast-out child make his fortune, or so it seemed to me. Obviously, I had not yet heard that the streets of New York were paved with gold" (Bettelheim, 1990, p. 133). In truth, it might be said that it was the streets of Chicago that were so paved for Bettelheim.

Overall, relatively few details about Bettelheim's childhood are available from a reading of his papers. He did write about regularly spending afternoons away from his family with an aunt, in order to escape an older intrusive, domineering sister and the authoritarian aspects of his parents ("Contemporaries: Bruno Bettelheim, Ph.D.," 1971). During this period of time, he reflected, he was probably more deeply influenced by the aunt than by his mother. He also refers to having had feelings of deep pessimism and problems related to depressive tendencies, which he associated with personal experiences within his family and adolescent turmoil, combined with the beginnings of World War I (Bettelheim, 1990). Those feelings appear to have been at least partly countered by an escape into reading, music and art, and the movies. But most of all, Bettelheim claimed, his adolescent years were marked by his readings of Freud and psychoanalysis from fourteen years of age on.

His own account of his introduction to psychoanalytic thinking is charming, but also may be instructive about an aspect of his personality during early adolescence and perhaps later. Bettelheim was part of a Viennese radical youth group, an important activity of which was regular Sunday outings to the Viennese woods. At one point, Bettelheim felt he was in danger of losing the interest of a girl with whom he was infatuated to an older boy (said to have been Otto Fenichel) who was discussing Freud's lectures with members of the group. Bettelheim spent the next week avidly immersed in psychoanalytic writings, the better to present himself on the following Sunday. In writing about this, Bettelheim acknowledged that his introduction to psychoanalysis was, thus, not the result of a wish to acquire a deeper knowledge about himself or mankind. Instead, his earliest interest stemmed from a narcissistic need to impress the girl and from competitive feelings toward the older boy. From another viewpoint, it illustrated a tendency to judge things by their peripheral appearances, that the girl was really more interested in what the other boy was saying than in him as a person. Nevertheless, Bettelheim claimed, "one week of complete concentration on psychoanalysis and I was hooked for life" (p. 127). However, it would be many years before his intellectual interest in psychoanalysis would become a deeper personal experience or a professional consideration for Bettelheim.

Dr. Bettelheim attended the University of Vienna for a number of years, during most of which he worked in the family business. He spent the first two years at the university studying German language and literature and the following two years studying philosophy, which he found too abstract for personal fulfillment. In 1928, he began a three-year psychoanalysis with Dr. Richard Sterba, prompted by feelings of inferiority and depression, related to a dislike of and boredom with the business world, indecisiveness about the aim of his studies at the university, and a crisis in his marriage. Two years later, he and his first wife (who was a teacher at the special school run by Anna Freud and Dorothy Burlingham) took into their home as a therapeutic experiment a mute seven-year old girl, who had previously been variously diagnosed as feeble-minded, brain damaged, and psychotic. Although the experiment may have contributed to the breakup of that marriage, it lasted until Hitler annexed Austria in 1938, at which time Mrs. Bettelheim and the girl left for America ("Contemporaries: Bruno Bettelheim, Ph.D.," 1971).

Some time prior to that, Bettelheim had once again changed his major at the University of Vienna to art history; he eventually focused on the area of aesthetics. Influenced by his experiences with psychoanalysis, he eventually wrote a dissertation that attempted to integrate the psychoanalytic perspective with a philosophical understanding of beauty (based largely on Kant), and he received his PhD from Vienna in 1937 or 1938, just before the *Anschluss* (Bettelheim, 1990). At that point, Bettelheim had undertaken an analysis, had demonstrated a real interest in helping emotionally disturbed youth, and had friends who had become psychoanalysts. There is no evidence, however, that he ever actually studied under Freud or that he ever was a member of any formal training group with Freud's students. Interestingly, though he began referring to himself as a psychoanalyst a few years after immigrating (Bettelheim, 1957), unlike some of his emigre colleagues, such as Rudolph Ekstein, he did not pursue formal psychoanalytic training in the United States, nor is it known that he really had private analytic patients.

Soon after the Nazi annexation of Austria, Bettelheim was arrested by the Gestapo, it has been said because of his underground activities in the social assistance section of the resistance movement against the Austrian Fascist government. He was first interned in Dachau, but shortly thereafter was transferred to Buchenwald, which is said to have been turned from an extermination camp into a working camp by the time of Bettelheim's arrival. Ernst Federn remembers, "At the time of Bettelheim's stay there, from September 1938 to April 1939, life was very bad indeed, but it was possible to survive, even for a person as unsuited to the practicalities of life as Bettelheim. He owes his survival to the chance of finding work in the stock-mending shop, where he could live in relative safety. He could also take advantage of the fact that he wore thick eyeglasses; for reasons I could never find out, the SS guards showed some respect for these" (Federn, 1990, p. 4).

The details of his release from Buchenwald in 1939 are unclear. However, shortly afterwards a Rockefeller grant enabled Ralph Tyler, then Chair of the Department of Education at the University of Chicago, to provide a position for Bettelheim as a research associate with the Progressive Education Association at Chicago, where he remained for two years. From 1942 to 1944, he was

Associate Professor of Psychology at Rockford College, Illinois, and then returned to the University of Chicago to become the principal, later director, of the Orthogenic School, which had been founded in 1913 as part of Rush Medical College. He remained as director of the Orthogenic School for three decades, and during that time he rose from the rank of assistant professor of educational psychology (1944) at the university, to full professor (1952), to the position of Stella M. Rowley distinguished service professor of education and professor of psychology and psychiatry (1963).

THE POLITICAL WRITINGS

Bettelheim arrived in the United States somewhat later in the process of escape and immigration of German intellectuals, artists, and academics. In 1933, Hitler had already begun a systematic exile of the academics, which eventually included 43 percent of all German academics, and 47 percent of the social scientists (Heilbut, 1984). As Heilbut has pointed out, "Such an extraordinary influx was bound to influence the American academy for decades: well into the 1970's, immigrants such as Karl Deutsch and Heinz Eulau in political science and Lewis Coser in sociology remained leaders of their disciplines, Eulau as president of the American Political Science Association and Coser as president of the American Sociological Association" (p. 75). The academic areas of art history and musicology were radically transformed by the immigrant scholars, who also became extremely influential in such other varied fields as existential philosophy and, in Bettelheim's case, psychoanalytic thought. Heilbut reminds us that in Europe, these scholars, "as the best heirs of Goethe, the last universal man, had constituted a society of polymaths" (p. 74). It followed that a large number of them, especially the younger intellectuals such as Bettelheim, initially achieved reputations in the United States as generalists. They jumped from one academic field to another, in a manner which would have compromised their reputations and chances for advancement in Europe, but which instead inspired academic admiration and success here.

Many of the immigrants completed some of their most important scholarly works at universities, such as the political philosophers Carl Friedrich at Harvard and Eric Voegelin at Louisiana State University. Much of the emigres' most productive work, however, was done in academic centers specifically set up for them, which also tended to reflect the ideological diversity of the various groups. These settings included the allegedly nonpolitical Institute for Advanced Study at Princeton, the activist and liberal University in Exile at the New School for Social Research, the leftist (somewhat Marxist) Institute for Social Research in New York, and Paul Lazerfield's more pragmatic, empirically oriented Bureau of Applied Social Research at Columbia University. In a relatively short period of time, the studies of unemployment, propaganda, prejudice, the decline of the family, and the impact of popular culture became refugee academic specialties, owing in part to the immigrants' earlier, painful experiences in Germany and Austria.

In time, the University of Chicago became the academic home for a number of brilliant immigrant scholars, who had previously been on the graduate faculty of the University in Exile at the New School. These scholars included Hans J. Morgenthau in international relations, Leo Strauss in political philosophy, and, somewhat later, Hanna Arendt in the field of social thought. Although Bettelheim had come directly to Chicago, his deep intellectual involvement with the New York academic immigrant interests and cultural debates became immediately evident in his earliest publications, which were specifically political in focus.

Bettelheim began to achieve notoriety in the United States after publishing "Individual and Mass Behavior in Extreme Situations" in 1943. Briefly, Bettelheim's article delineated four stages in the process of adaptation to the camp situation, beginning with the initial shock of being unlawfully imprisoned and concluding with the prisoner adapting himself to life in the camp. He described the different categories of prisoners, as well as the prisoner class system within the camp, which he would more fully elaborate in his later paper, "The Concentration Camp as a Class State" (Bettelheim 1947). He attempted to understand his observations of himself and other prisoners' behaviors in the camp in terms of the major psychological defense mechanisms, which included dissociation and a regression to infantile or childlike behavior patterns and defenses.

The latter included a growing ambivalence toward their families (related to magical thinking or wishes that if nothing changed in the outside world, they would not be changed by the camp experience either). Bitter reactions to changes in their families seemed, for Bettelheim, to be a form of reaction formation against the growing realization that they were, in fact, changing.

Other aspects of the regression into infantile behavior included despondency and finding satisfaction in daydreaming, rather than in action. Childlike behavior was fostered by special guard techniques, such as the strict regulation of defecation and forcing prisoners to say "thou" to one another, used then in Germany only among small children. They were forced to perform nonsensical tasks, which encouraged feelings of debasement at having to do such childish and stupid labor. Prisoners lived totally in the present, losing a sense of sequential time, and they became unable to establish durable object relations with other prisoners.

In the final stage of adjustment to the camp situation, according to Bettelheim, the prisoner's personality changed so fundamentally as to accept as his own the values of the Gestapo, and identification with the aggressor became a major mechanism. In individual and group daydreams about life after release from camp, the longer a prisoner had been in camp, the more distorted were his fantasies. The fantasies of the older prisoners often took the form of "messianic hopes," beliefs that out of this ordeal they would emerge as the future leaders of Germany, if not the world. Concluding his study, Bettelheim suggested that the study of the Nazi methods used to break down prisoners' personalities might one day lead to the development of techniques to rehabilitate those who were unable to function as autonomous and self-reliant persons, an enterprise he was to undertake a year later at the Orthogenic School.

Ernst Federn has stated that this paper reported observations that were made in conversations between himself, Bettelheim, and a Dr. Brief, who of the three was the only fully trained psychoanalyst (Federn, 1990). In his paper, however, Bettelheim claimed that the observations derived solely from his own investigation, undertaken in part to protect himself from a disintegration of his personality. He said that he tried to check his conclusions with other prisoners, but could find only two who were trained and interested enough to participate. According to Bettelheim, these were Alfred Fischer, M.D., and an unnamed participant (perhaps Federn), who was still at Buchenwald in 1943.

The concentration camp experience was to continue as a haunting interest in Bettelheim's writings throughout his life. In a 1971 interview, Dr. Bettelheim alluded in a somewhat puzzling parable to what may have been an important aspect of that persisting interest:

> Three men are mountain climbing. One falls into a crevice, but he is still alive. Of the other two, one must go for help with the remaining man standing by the crevice until that help arrives. But of these other two, one says that he cannot stay by the crevice, which may well be an all-night, subzero ordeal, and without waiting to see whether the other agrees to his all-night vigil, he runs off for help. Well, fortunately, everybody came out of this situation safely. But it unalterably changed the life of the man who went for help. He had to face the fact that when the chips were down, he had found himself wanting. [Contemporaries: Bruno Bettelheim, Ph.D., 1971, p. 31]

While this simple story may relate to a real-life mountain climbing experience, as a metaphor it might also more generally reflect Bettelheim's feelings about his release from the concentration camp. The parable can be contrasted with Bettelheim's assessment of Dr. Janusz Korczak in his final book of essays (Bettelheim, 1990). Bettelheim proclaimed that Korczak was a righteous martyr, because he had rejected many offers to be saved from extermination in the death camps in order not to desert the orphaned children to whose well-being he had devoted his life in the Warsaw ghetto. Taken together, these two sets of comments may suggest that Bettelheim experienced strong, enduring feelings of ambivalence and guilt about his own release and having to leave others behind. From this point of view, one might speculate that Bettelheim's frequent criticisms of Jewish prisoner behaviors and his delight in demolishing cultural cliches, such as the near-sainthood of Anne Frank, were related in part to an attempt to deal with the more conflictual feelings associated with his own release. In this sense, the criticism functioned to deidealize the prisoners left behind and to provide a defensive distancing from them. But while Bettelheim viewed his arguments about the prisoners and camp life as being based upon more realistic objectivity, his protagonists viewed them as unempathic devaluations of the prisoners by a man who should have understood their ordeal well.

Among the arguments which many found controversial, if not objectionable, were Bettelheim's descriptions of social classes within the camps, where, he claimed, the prisoner aristocracy lost all empathy with the fate, the feeling and thinking, the experiences and suffering of lower-class prisoners. According to Bettelheim, the prisoner aristocracy controlled and suppressed the majority of the prisoners, for the SS in order to exercise a protective function for themselves (Bettelheim, 1947). He dismissed any attempt to glorify the few hundred prisoners at Treblinka who finally revolted against the camp guards, stoically observing that he could not "accept it as sufficient cause for pride that of eight hundred thousand prisoners who passively went to their death at Treblinka, only the very last thousand, and only when their death was imminent, finally tried to break out of [that] human slaughterhouse" (Bettelheim, 1967b, p. 23).

He described a central aspect of what he viewed as Jewish "ghetto mentality," a sense of martyrdom, as a major reason for the failure of the Jews to have revolted earlier: "To the ghetto Jew individual destiny counts for nothing. So it really doesn't matter how many millions get killed, or by whom. All that counts is that martyrdom which is a symbol of the destiny of the Jewish people" (Bettelheim, 1967b, p. 30). In an earlier article on Jewish ghetto thinking, Bettelheim clearly placed a large part of the blame on the Jewish people themselves, who he felt exhibited procrastination in the face of their annihilation, refused to part with their fortunes and possessions in order to escape, failed to provide financial help to poorer Jews for passage out, and fell back upon either pervasive feelings of resignation or the ingrained habit of believing that ultimately the ghetto oppressor would relent (Bettelheim, 1960). Accordingly, Bettelheim strongly objected to *The Diary of Anne Frank* (1952) for the reception it received as a glorification of helpless Jewish passivity, ignoring what he saw as the real lesson of that story, which was how denial hastened the destruction of the Frank family (Bettelheim, 1960). Bettelheim, the former victim, had become the judge, but unfortunately, some felt, he was at times almost as harsh a judge of the Jewish people as of the Nazi oppressors.

Returning to the time of Bettelheim's first publication in 1943, it is instructive not simply to note that Bettelheim's first publication quickly established a notoriety which grew with his subsequent political commentaries, but also to attempt to trace how the initial notoriety occurred. The different immigrant academic centers were described briefly earlier, and it was pointed out that they tended to represent differing, inclusive political cliques. For example, the New School's immigrant faculty tended to be respectable academic and political veterans, while the Institute for Social Research, which had been founded in Germany as the Frankfurt Institute, attracted leftist intellectuals, including Walter Benjamin, Paul Tillich, Adorno, Marcuse, and Erich Fromm. While other immigrant academic centers were frequently concerned with practical matters such as unemployment, propaganda, and empirical sociological analysis, psychoanalysis and art were the early predominant interests for the institute members, who promoted the work of some of the most difficult of the modernists, such as Schoenberg and Samuel Beckett (Heilbut, 1984).

Academically, sociology was one of the most exciting and energized fields, with ongoing debates between the differing views and methodological approaches of Paul Lazerfield at the Bureau of Applied Social Research at Columbia, Karl Mannheim at the New School, and Adorno and Otto Horkheimer at the Institute for Social Research. The institute was known for its sharp interest in class relations and for a pessimistic view of the impact of mass culture on the individual. Bettelheim's 1943 study of the concentration camps, arguing that Fascism produced something similar to a psychological collapse, seemed to parallel the Frankfurters' view of the effects of mass culture in general. Further, other factors contributed to the institute's members' strong interest in Bettelheim's article: its tone was both sociological and psychoanalytic, its author's previous training had been in art history and aesthetics, and its publication came just at the time that the institute members were discovering the advantages of taking a more visible public stand against Fascism.

In 1944, the institute offered a very well-attended series on National Socialism, and Bettelheim's study was afforded both credibility and a wider audience when it was presented as the subject of the final lecture in the series. Bettelheim's public association with this powerful academic clique would last at least until the mid-1950s, as evidenced then by his contribution to a major German sociological anthology, which otherwise included only the Frankfurt group of sociology academics (Bettelheim, 1955a).

In 1944, the institute began a series of studies focusing on prejudice, with financial support from the American Jewish Committee. The studies were planned to incorporate the latest methodology in data analysis and psychoanalytic explanation, and Bettelheim was invited to collaborate on that research project. The results of his studies on prejudice, undertaken with the sociologist Morris Janowitz, were later presented in a number of publications, including: "Ethnic Tolerance: A Function of Social and Personal Control" (Bettelheim and Janowitz, 1949), "Reactions to Fascist Propaganda—A Pilot Study" (Bettelheim and Janowitz, 1950b), "Prejudice" (Bettelheim, 1950b), and *Dynamics of Prejudice* (Bettelheim and Janowitz, 1950a). While there can be no doubt of the need for careful studies of ethnic prejudice, nor of the integrity of Bettelheim's intentions, a closer examination of those studies raises serious questions about the validity and applicability of their conclusions. The initial study of ethnic tolerance and intolerance among World War II veterans was described as "an account of a significant statistical study of racial discrimination" (Bettelheim, 1950b) and speculated that the study aimed "to throw light on the principles of group hostility in general and on ethnic hostility as a special subtype" (Bettelheim and Janowitz, 1949, p. 137).

The first study concluded that neither age, education, religion, political affiliation, income, nor social status seemed to account for significant differences in the degree or nature of intolerance. The major finding of the initial study of prejudice or ethnic intolerance was that an acceptance of the major institutions of social control or external authority (such as the Veterans Administration, the political party system, the federal government, and the economic system) seemed to facilitate tolerance of some minorities. However, a review of this study leads to the conclusion that it was seriously flawed in terms of generally accepted research methodology. First, the sample was said to be randomly selected; however, it was not a representative sample, but instead was restricted to 150 male enlisted men, who were all from lower-and lower-middle-class backgrounds. Moreover, members of a number of major ethnic groups were excluded from the study group. Homogeneous samples, such as this, usually result in lower correlation, reliability, and validity coefficients, since most variance would represent error or unknown factors. Second, an attempt was made to apply content analysis to the free-association responses of the subjects. However, the content analysis was not the more rigorous quasi-experimental type, but rather appears to have been largely a selection of subjects' comments to illustrate the authors' hypotheses. Finally, while psychoanalytic terminology was introduced to (or grafted onto) the study in an attempt to strengthen and broaden the findings, it is clear that the conclusions should not have been generalized to the general population.

Soon after the first investigation, Bettelheim and Janowitz conducted a related study of reactions to exposure to Fascist propaganda, drawing their subjects from the restricted sample of the first study (Bettelheim and Janowitz, 1950b). The resulting sample was even more limited than the first, with the number of participants dwindling from 150 to 33. In the original publication from the second study, no statistical evidence of significance was presented, and much of the argument was based upon anecdotal accounts of selected responses by participants. As with the prior study, untested heuristic psychological descriptions were introduced, seeming to give the appearance of a more general credibility to the findings, when in fact it suffered from even greater sample limitations than the initial research. Bettelheim and Janowitz concluded, nevertheless, that their second study confirmed the main conclusion of their larger earlier study.

One of the most interesting observations about Bettelheim's conclusions was that while his sponsors (the members of the Institute for Social Research) disdained the effects of mass culture, Bettelheim ended up contending that a cure for the problem of prejudice was to be found in the establishment of social consensus and an acceptance of authority. Unlike Adorno (Horkheimer and Adorno, 1972), he seemed to strongly link tolerance with the influence of social conformity (Heilbut, 1984). Somewhat later, however, Bettelheim made a strong distinction between what he saw as the need for an acceptance of authority and his perception of the detrimental effects of "mass society" (Bettelheim, 1955a).

A DARKER CHAPTER:
WRITINGS ON THE VIETNAM WAR PROTESTORS

The theme of authority would later reemerge vehemently in Bettelheim's writings about student protests during the Vietnam era, and much of what he had to say aroused heated controversy amongst those who opposed the United States' involvement in that war (Bettelheim, 1969b, 1972). Rereading these writings from the retrospective vantage point of some twenty years can leave one with the sense that the war protesters aroused in Bettelheim strong, almost overpowering memories of the rise of Hitler Germany. He responded to the protest activities by attacking the anti-Vietnam war movement with a series of arguments, which were frequently framed in psychoanalytic terms.

His arguments took a variety of turns, beginning with a flippant dismissal of millions of Americans' strongly held convictions against involvement in the war in Vietnam. To the charge that the war was immoral, Bettelheim simply countered that "all wars are immoral." Moreover, Bettelheim continued, "what youth is fighting against is not so much the war in Viet Nam or the global balance, but an America whose technology seems to have robbed them of any place in the real work of the world" (Bettelheim, 1969b, p. 32). The turmoil of youth was seen by Bettelheim in a paradoxical way: on the one hand, he stated that the turmoil of young people is "an age phenomenon which is natural" and which has existed since ancient times (Bettelheim, 1972). However, when more convenient to his arguments against the war protesters, he seemed to shift to a belief that adolescent revolt is *not* a natural stage, but rather is a relatively new phenomenon precipitated by the inherent evils of technology, a decline in the quality of family relationships, and the negative side-effects of affluence in the modern industrial state (Bettelheim, 1969b).

Bettelheim characterized the war protesters and their antiwar movement as the "Fascism of the Left," a label which was related to his belief that there were strong similarities between the American protest activities and the political movements which characterized pre-Hitler and Hitler Germany. The seeming parallels between the war protesters and the Nazis, according to Bettelheim, included: a fascination with violent revolution against "the establishment," an anti-intellectual stance, the reliance upon a simplistic reduction of complex issues, the protesters' self-definition as the "true believers," and ultimately, for Bettelheim, the symbolic student "takeovers" at a number of major American universities (Bettelheim, 1969b).

In the end, however, Bettelheim reduced the beliefs and actions of the war protesters simply to behavioral manifestations of emotional disturbance. As evidence, he cited his own interpretations of protesters' statements in the news media and limited clinical case material. With reference to the latter, Bettelheim's descriptions made the source and type of treatment ambiguous. It was written to sound as though the material came from his private therapeutic or analytic treatment of patients, although to my knowledge it did not. Nevertheless, from that limited case material, Bettelheim generalized that what was true for two therapy patients was generally characteristic for most, if not all members of the antiwar movement. Accordingly, radical political activity was portrayed as a desperate attempt to escape severe depression and to avoid complete breaks with reality. For Bettelheim, who at times appeared to be somewhat enthralled with the concept of authority, resolution of the protest situation, and youth turmoil in general, was to be found more in the reestablishment of a greater authority within the family unit and by university administrations, than in the correction of any particular social inequities.

Bettelheim's articles about the protesters were not submitted for scrutiny to established, refereed academic journals. Instead, they appeared in popularized political magazines with a more general readership. At about the same time, a lengthy statement of his position against the antiwar movement was presented before the Congressional Special Subcommittee on Education and was entered into the Congressional Record, with Congressman Pucinski's introduction interpreting Bettelheim's arguments as that "Dr. Bettelheim has called our attention to the fact that some of those participating in campus disorders are emotionally disturbed and in need of professional help in the treatment of their personal problems" (Pucinski, 1969, p. E2473).

CLINICAL WRITINGS
ON MILIEU TREATMENT

Just as Bettelheim's early political writings had been facilitated by his involvement in a politically oriented, intellectual clique (the immigrant scholars composing New York's Institute for Social Research), so his early writings about the treatment of disturbed children were deeply influenced by his dialogues and collaborations with a small circle of clinicians, which included Fritz Redl and the psychoanalyst Emmy Sylvester. Although Bettelheim's clinical writings were initiated somewhat later than his political ones, after 1947 a flurry of publishing activity was apparent, with at least eight major clinical articles appearing between 1947 and 1949. The majority of those early articles focused in one way or another on the concept of milieu therapy and, in particular, on its application with emotionally disturbed children at the Orthogenic School of the University of Chicago (Bettelheim, 1948a,b, 1949; Bettelheim and Sylvester, 1947, 1948, 1949a,b, 1950).

Bettelheim acknowledged that milieu therapy was not a new psychotherapeutic technique. He noted that Anna Freud had considered it earlier, although with skepticism, as an adjunct for some cases of child analysis, and that August Aichorn had been optimistic about the therapeutic potential of a carefully arranged institutional setting. Fritz Redl was also publishing a number of articles about the use of special milieu therapy techniques with disturbed children (Redl, 1942, 1943, 1944, 1949; Redl and Wineman, 1951, 1952). A major emphasis in Redl's writings was on developing for staff members methods of behavioral control, techniques for interview interventions in the milieu, and strategies for maintaining the structure or framework of the milieu. At the Orthogenic School, however, the structure or framework of the milieu was assumed–it rested significantly upon the presence of Bettelheim as the autocratic director of the school. Accordingly, the emphasis of Bettelheim's writing about the milieu was largely on describing the effects of an already existent cohesive, nonchaotic therapeutic environment on the emotional process of rehabilitation through a variety of illustrations from case material, rather than on the specification of practical strategies for maintaining the stability of a therapeutic setting. Nevertheless, that Bettelheim was following the work of Aichorn (1935) and Redl is clear both from his early emphasis on the effect of the milieu and from his interest in the treatment of delinquents (Bettelheim, 1948a,b, 1949, 1955b; Bettelheim and Sylvester, 1949a,b, 1950). In this context, Bettelheim discussed the appropriateness of closed versus open treatment institutions for delinquents (Bettelheim, 1948a), the delinquent's concern for and confusion about moral issues (Bettelheim and Sylvester, 1950), and somatic symptoms which develop in children as they begin to give up their delinquent, tension discharging patterns of behavior (Bettelheim, 1948b; Bettelheim and Sylvester, 1949b).

In terms of milieu therapy, Bettelheim's initial writings attempted to specify some of the beneficial group effects of milieu treatment upon the individual child (Bettelheim and Sylvester, 1947), to describe some of the general characteristics of and indications for milieu treatment (Bettelheim and Sylvester, 1948, 1949a), and to distinguish between a therapeutic "home," psychiatric treatment center, and the psychiatric school (Bettelheim, 1949). With regard to the general characteristics of a therapeutic milieu, Bettelheim repeatedly emphasized the need, applied in ways particular to each child, for an almost unconditional gratification of the child's basic needs, a secure and protective setting, and carefully measured dosages of reality. Milieu therapy was indicated both for children whose ability to maintain contact with parental figures had been catastrophically destroyed and for those children who apparently had not acquired the tools for establishing such a relationship in the first place (Bettelheim and Sylvester, 1949a). Thus, according to Bettelheim, milieu therapy was most indicated where the basic needs of the child had been so neglected that the child lacked psychological integration at even the pregenital level. For children who had achieved a higher level of integration, psychotherapy alone might be indicated, for example, in situations where a disturbance in the Oedipal phase occasioned a regression to earlier developmental stages as a point of fixation. In such instances, Bettelheim felt, an interpersonal relationship with the psychotherapist could be expected to resolve the prior traumatization. It should be noted, however, that a reading of Bettelheim's early papers suggests that a number of children at the Orthogenic School during that period of time did not primarily display the deeper pregenital lack of psychological integration, which he demarcated as the special province of residential milieu treatment.

Finally, in his remarks distinguishing the characteristics of a psychiatric school from either a therapeutic group home or a psychiatric treatment center, Bettelheim clarified what he viewed as important differences between individual psychiatric treatment and milieu care (Bettelheim, 1949). First, he pointed out that the prevalent psychiatric techniques had been developed in treating adults, concentrating on uncovering the repressed and changing deviate personality structures. However, Bettelheim believed that for those children most in need of residential milieu treatment, emotional difficulties stemmed from their basic inability to organize their personalities in the first place and from a near absence of repressive defensive mechanisms. According to Bettelheim, "the psychiatric school's therapeutic task is to bring order into chaos rather than to reorganize a deviately put together cosmos" (Bettelheim, 1949, p. 91). In other words, whereas psychiatric treatment often aimed toward permitting greater instinctual gratification by lifting repression, the education of the psychiatric school strives more toward the socialization of wild, overpowering instinctual tendencies.

Second, the prevalent schools of psychiatry relied upon the transference relationship and its exploration as the major tool, presupposing the previous existence of important relationships, feelings about which could be transferred onto the therapist. In Bettelheim's view, however, children needing milieu treatment characteristically had experienced no relationships which were suitable as a vehicle for transference. Accordingly, the psychiatric school needed to be concerned with helping the child order the world of the present, while psychiatric treatment was seen as more concerned with doing away with misinterpretations of past experiences. In Bettelheim's milieu setting, "instead of reliving the pathogenic past, the child is helped to live successfully in the present. Convincing demonstrations of ego strength thus take the place of speculation about the possible sources of its weaknesses" (Bettelheim, 1949, p. 93). This view that psychotic patients cannot effect transference relationships, since they cannot cathect representations of external objects, has been challenged by other writers (Arlow and Brenner, 1969). According to them, the transferences "may be transient, volatile, unstable, and fraught with aggression, but they represent, nonetheless, the same fundamental process which can be recognized in the transference of neurotic patients . . . " (Arlow and Brenner, 1969, p.8). Further, Bettelheim's assertion that psychotic children in residential care are incapable of transference relationships disregards the existence of their transference reactions to the institution itself, although his early anecdotal writings do illustrate the presence of such displacements.

Nevertheless, despite Bettelheim's arguments that individual psychotherapy had little to offer for children in need of residential treatment, such treatment was in fact provided to some children at the Orthogenic School. For example, one of the earliest examples of the richly detailed case studies of children at the school is clearly based on insights derived from a boy's individual psychotherapy sessions with Dr. Emmy Sylvester (Bettelheim and Sylvester, 1950). The clarity and persuasiveness of that study's narrative style was later to become characteristic of Bettelheim's writings about schizophrenic and autistic children, those best known to the general public including, "Schizophrenic Art: A Case Study" (Bettelheim, 1952), "Joey: A 'Mechanical Boy'"(Bettelheim, 1959); and "Laurie" (Bettelheim, 1969a). Bettelheim's more general comments about both the type of pathology and kind of treatment solely indicated by residential care seem somewhat contradictory when viewed in terms of his practical descriptions of the Orthogenic School. This contrast points out Bettelheim's tendency to be dramatic and to describe situations in their extremes, while practice reveals that gradations are the rule.

CONCENTRATION CAMP REACTIONS
AND CHILDHOOD SCHIZOPHRENIA

Within two years, Bettelheim would temporarily shift the major thrust of his writings away from delinquency and the general aspects of the therapeutic milieu, concentrating more on describing the backgrounds and treatment of schizophrenic and autistic children. The connection between this shift and Bettelheim's concentration camp experiences is vividly illustrated by one of his most poignant articles on childhood schizophrenia, "Schizophrenia as a Reaction.to Extreme Situations" (Bettelheim, 1956), which was, of course, only a slight variation of the title of his original 1943 commentary on the disintegrative psychological effects of the Nazi internment. Bettelheim asserted that an important similarity between the two situations was "that the youngster who develops childhood schizophrenia seems to feel about himself and his life exactly as the concentration camp prisoner felt about his, namely, that he is totally at the mercy of irrational forces which are bent on using him for their goals, irrespective of his" (Bettelheim, 1956, p. 512). Thus, Bettelheim claimed, "the psychological cause of childhood schizophrenia is the child's subjective feeling of living permanently in an extreme situation . . . helpless in the face of threats to his very life, at the mercy of insensitive powers which are motivated only by their own incomprehensible whims, and of being deprived of any interpersonal, need-satisfying relationship" (Bettelheim, 1956, p. 513).

Further, Bettelheim felt that there was a strong parallel between schizophrenic reactions among the prisoners and the symptoms associated with autism and schizophrenia in children. In particular, both the psychological devastation precipitated by the concentration camp experience and the symptomatology of childhood schizophrenia appeared to be, for Bettelheim, the consequence of a massive regression (Bettelheim, 1956). Finally, Bettelheim's study of the camp prisoners' experiences led him to agree with speculation that a milieu constructed as the *opposite* of the camp environment could facilitate significant psychological rehabilitation, pointing out another author's conclusion that "if one has seen how the prisoners experienced utter deterioration when exposed to such conditions and how quickly they regain their human qualities after liberation, once they feel assured of relative security and adequate food, one gains some inkling of what a world could be like in which every human being had absolute assurance that his life and needs would be guaranteed by the social structure instead of being endangered by it" (Bettelheim, 1947, p. 637).

On the surface, Bettelheim's analogy seems persuasive, but closer examination reveals at least two important limitations. First, Bettelheim's commentary on the prisoners' behaviors seems to exaggerate and overstate pathology. He suggested a general regression to formal schizophrenic states in the camp population, with "startling" exceptions, when such a total, true clinical regression may actually have occurred only in certain predisposed cases. In contrast, Edith Jacobson's (1949, 1959) more clinically refined studies of regression and depersonalization observed in a group of female political prisoners in Nazi Germany reached far less dogmatic conclusions. Whereas Bettelheim stressed the pathological dimension of prisoners' regressive reactions to external trauma and tended to extend the pathological diagnosis as characteristic of the entire prisoner population, Jacobson more clearly distinguished the more transient infantile regressions and resultant ego defensive depersonalization seen in the more numerous psychologically normal prisoners, from the more serious and entrenched reactions of neurotic prisoners. Accordingly, she cautioned that although her comments attempted to describe certain common regressive ego defenses among the prisoners, her study did not explore "the true psychopathology of prison confinement." In fact, she pointed out that the more severe syndromes of prison psychosis were not seen in the group of political prisoners she observed. A second limitation to Bettelheim's analogy between the reactions of the concentration camp prisoners and schizophrenic children involves the differing basic underlying mechanisms of those two differing situations. The reactions of the prisoners were generally under the dominance of regression as the main force instituting a partial backward movement to earlier developmental points. However, with schizophrenic children, who are characterized by severe pregenital disturbances, major fixations tend to play a much more dominant role than the defensive mechanism of regression (Greenacre, 1960).

THOUGHTS ON REGRESSION

Nevertheless, regression became a concept of pivotal importance in Bettelheim's earlier, widely published case study presentations of the psychological rehabilitation of schizophrenic and autistic children in residential milieu treatment at the Orthogenic School (Bettelheim, 1952, 1959, 1969). However, when Bettelheim discussed the underlying processes of the pregenital childhood schizophrenic disturbances, he tended to commingle the concepts of fixation and regression–sometimes the child never achieved a sense of autonomy, at other times the child's development receded from a perceived autonomy in the face of extreme trauma. It was only when talking about the actual course of treatment for the schizophrenic or autistic child that Bettelheim appeared to focus more clearly upon his understanding of regression, in particular a concept of "regression as progression." Specifically, he claimed that "quite a number of schizophrenic children, at the crucial point in their rehabilitation when they're ready to reintegrate their personalities, . . . begin their new life symbolically; so much so, that they undergo again the experience of being reborn" (Bettelheim, 1956, p. 518).

In case studies published during this period (Bettelheim, 1952, 1956, 1969), Bettelheim described regressions as crucial points in the treatment process of three children who he claimed were autistic: one involved a regression to infantile behavior which he interpreted as an attempt at "rebirth," and the two others manifested symbolic womb and rebirth fantasies. However, rather than elaborate more fully on the nature of that notion of regression as a significant turning point in the course of treatment, Bettelheim initially deferred that discussion to another time, stating abruptly that "unfortunately, presentation of the evidence on this process of rebirth would transgress the limitations of space" (Bettelheim, 1956, p. 518). Ten years later, he did return to a consideration of this topic, when he presented expanded versions of those three early case studies in *The Empty Fortress* (1967a). Unfortunately, even this later presentation of his understanding of regression was a disappointingly limited one. Bettelheim's admittedly "nontechnical" explanation of his understanding of regression in the crucial phase of treatment was limited to the temporal sense of regression, "a recapturing of early experience through a partial reexperience that will support a very different development" (p. 292). Even were one to assume that the treatment of schizophrenic children could be characterized by the predominance of such regression, the paucity of Bettelheim's account of it stands in stark contrast to the much more detailed examination of the many types and varied dynamics of regression by other writers at that time (Jacobson, 1959; Greenacre, 1960; A. Freud, 1963, 1965, 1966; Arlow and Brenner, 1969; Jackson, 1969).

In particular, Bettelheim seemed to understand both the wish to reexperience the womb and the wish to be reborn as one form of adaptive regression, namely, the wish to start all over again in order to enjoy a new and better life. Marcovitz (1952) had written earlier about children presenting fantasies of rebirth in the course of therapy as an example of the illusory deja vu experience. According to Marcovitz, such experiences represent a regressive wish for union with the mother, both Oedipal and preoedipal. In agreement with Bettelheim, he further interpreted the rebirth fantasy as the wish to retrieve the past and to start over again in the face of feelings of disappointment. Arlow's (1959) paper on the structure of the deja vu experience examines it as a reassuring, transitory defensive regression of a specific ego function, namely, the sense of reality. According to Arlow, "The wish for a second chance is apparently a subsidiary motive in the structure of the deja vu experience, not essential in its organization and clearly secondary to the defensive need of the ego to ward off the anxiety which threatens to emerge when the structure of a current situation stimulates and symbolizes quite precisely an important, unconscious conflict associated with concrete experiences from the past" (p. 625).

As mentioned earlier, Bettelheim seemed to understand both the womb and rebirth fantasies as one phenomenon, which he interpreted upward as the wish for a second chance. Freud (1918), however, had distinguished more clearly between the two fantasies in his discussion of an infantile neurosis, and interpreted them more deeply in terms of infantile sexual wishes. For Freud, while the notion of being born again to a happier life was an agreeable enough thought, he believed that the womb and rebirth fantasies demanded a more rigorous interpretation than simply that of the second chance. Accordingly, Freud proposed:

> The former, the womb-phantasy, is frequently derived . . . from an attachment to the father. There is a wish to be inside the mother's womb in order to replace her during coitus–in order to take her place in regard to the father. The phantasy of rebirth, on the other hand, is in all probability regularly a softened substitute (a euphemism, one might say) for the phantasy of incestuous intercourse with the mother. . . . Thus the two phantasies are revealed as one another's counterparts: they give expression, according as the subject's attitude is feminine or masculine, to his wish for sexual intercourse with his father or with his mother. [p. 583]

Thus, while an understanding of the concept of regression has always been considered important in classical psychoanalytic theory, Bettelheim seemed to display certain semantic confusions about that psychological process, tended to avoid a clear and detailed explanation of what he understood by regression, and relied upon a relatively simplified reification of that clinical concept. This was somewhat characteristic of Bettelheim's writings about other theoretical concepts. It suggests that he tended to be much more invested in developing a compelling, though often rhetorical explanation of the everyday practical treatment in his milieu setting, than he was in establishing a theoretically cohesive groundwork for his observations. Finally, while it cannot be denied that the topic of regression is an immensely difficult and complicated one for anyone to examine in depth, Bettelheim may have been impelled by more personal reasons to focus on the womb and rebirth fantasies in treatment, but to deal with them, and with regression in general, in only a relatively cursory manner. First, Bettelheim's focus probably reflected his great personal sense of hopefulness about disturbed children and his belief in the power of that hope in treatment, although he may not always have recognized the dangers of over-emphasizing it. Second, Bettelheim saw a striking parallel between his observations of the dominant preoccupation of concentration camp prisoners' daydreams of starting a new life after their release and the fantasies of rebirth which seemed to emerge at an important point in the treatment of schizophrenic children. In Bettelheim's view, only those prisoners "who managed really to begin, in a fashion, a new life after their release fully overcame the damaging influence of the camps" (Bettelheim, 1956, p. 517). It is important, then, to consider that to some extent, what Bettelheim was beholding in his work with children was both shaped and limited by an important aspect of his own experience. Specifically, it was during this period of his life that he was, in fact, undergoing a form of the rebirth process himself, reinventing himself anew and transforming himself in the eyes of the public from a 'Viennese upper–middle-class businessman to a self-trained "psychoanalyst."

PARENTAL BLAME AND OTHER CONTROVERSIES

While it is beyond the scope of this paper to further examine Bettelheim's early writings on childhood psychosis in depth, many are aware that Bettelheim's approach and conclusions have been heatedly debated. Foremost, with regard to genuinely autistic children, it is now commonly accepted that psychoanalytic milieu therapy is not the indicated treatment. Second, Bettelheim's stress on a detailed elaboration of the configurations of what he believed to be the historical antecedents of a child's pathology, some felt, obscured what really went on in treatment. This difficulty in pinpointing what were actually the most effective influences in the actual treatment situation was not helped by Bettelheim's attitude that *everything* was important, that it was the whole, cohesive milieu which counted in terms of effectiveness. A third major issue was related to Bettelheim's views about the mother's role in the development of childhood schizophrenia. When speaking more generally about the beginnings of childhood psychosis, Bettelheim stated:

> Returning to the problem of the origin of childhood schizo-
> phrenia, it can be said that the mother's pathology is often
> severe. . . . But this proves neither that these mothers created
> the schizophrenic process, nor that specifics of their patholo-
> gies explain those of the children. It seems that the concentra-
> tion on the mother, or the mother-child relation, is the conse-

quence of an unrealistic ideal–that of the perfect infant-mother symbiosis. . . . We have overlooked the fact that individuation, and with it stress and pain, begins at birth. Fortunately, this is being recognized, and psychoanalysts now decry the haunting image of the rejecting mother. [Bettelheim, 1956, p. 511]

However, Bettelheim's stress on historical antecedents, accompanied by the conclusion that a regressive reinstitution of a state of primary narcissism must of necessity have been conditioned by some trauma in the very earliest months of life, unfortunately led his particular case study reconstructions to almost conclusively lay the blame for children's emotional disturbances upon the parents, and specifically upon the mother, or the so-called schizophrenogenic mother (Arlow and Brenner, 1969).

Additional problems raised by his articles include an almost unbounded, iconoclastic optimism about the possibility of successfully treating severe disturbances, coupled with inflated success-rate claims and a lack of rigorous follow-up studies to document the effectiveness of his methods (Zimmerman and Sanders, 1988). This overzealousness was especially evident, though fortunately in a more limited area, when Bettelheim turned his interest to the treatment of psychosomatic disturbances. Unlike Greenacre (1960), who referred to that part of psychoanalytic research as "the unpruned crop of psychosomatic studies," Bettelheim enthusiastically embraced the notion of a psychological basis for somatic problems, with little sense of discrimination. Accordingly, Bettelheim claimed that all manner of sometimes long-standing physical and somatic difficulties, including clumsiness, allergies, asthmatic attacks, dermatitis, athlete's foot, ringworm, warts, poor hearing, and visual defects, disappeared spontaneously under the influence of the therapeutic milieu of the Orthogenic School (Bettelheim, 1948b; Bettelheim and Sylvester, 1949a,b).

BOOKS ABOUT THE ORTHOGENIC SCHOOL

A generally popular reception for Bettelheim's articles and case studies was followed by the publication of a number of books based upon his work at the Orthogenic School, including: *Love Is Not Enough* (1950a), *Truants from Life* (1955b), *The Empty Fortress* (1967a), and *A Home for the Heart* (1974). A brief summary of that body of work (Zimmerman, 1990) has described *Love Is Not Enough* as Bettelheim's effort to detail the principles of a therapeutic milieu in the residential treatment context, through a discussion of the events of everyday life in the care of the severely disturbed children at the school. In *Truants from Life*, Bettelheim shifted his focus from the details of the overall milieu, to a presentation of four case studies, which illustrated the histories and treatments of different childhood disturbances: psychosis, anorexia, institutionalism, and delinquency. *The Empty Fortress* extended this exploration of childhood psychopathology and gave a lengthy presentation of the efforts at the Orthogenic School to treat the most severe form of childhood psychosis, infantile autism, with three children.

In his final major work on the school, *A Home for the Heart*, Bettelheim returned to his initial theme of the overall therapeutic milieu, this time told largely through the experiences of the staff members. In a sense, this work also represented an attempt to provide a systemic evaluation of the school's milieu, initially elaborated by Henry (1957). Ironically, although Bettelheim insisted on calling the Orthogenic School a psychiatric *school* rather than a treatment center, most of his works dealt largely with the emotional life and dormitory experiences of the school's children and adolescents. Sanders's recent volume on the school, *A Greenhouse for the Mind* (1989), has focused specifically, for the first time, on the educational experiences and cognitive development of youth at the school.

A CERTAIN SADNESS OF THE LATER YEARS

Upon retirement from the Orthogenic School, Dr. Bettelheim relocated to California, where he continued to write. In 1976, he published *The Uses of Enchantment*, which initially was widely praised both for its psychoanalytic interpretations of fairy tales and for the compelling arguments in support of the importance of them for children (Bettelheim, 1976). From an academic perspective, however, a recent scholarly review of Bettelheim's psychoanalytic presentation has revealed serious mistakes and flaws, resulting from his many failures to consult and cite existent research in the field (Dundes, 1991). The degree of carelessness pointed out by Dundes suggests that an intellectual fascination with the psychological meaning of fairy tales was not the only strong motivating force at work for Bettelheim. For example, when speculatively taken at a more personal level, Bettelheim's strong recommendations of European folk tales for children may also be viewed as a reflection of his own growing sense of homesickness for the old country, an indication that his earlier affirmation of traditional American values as a spectacular improvement over the foibles of European romantics and Marxists was beginning to falter (Heilbut, 1984). Heilbut reported that when a group of Californians questioned the unrealistic happy endings of fairy tales, Bettelheim exploded, "Leave me at peace with your reality. It comes out of my ears. Your children are so thick they will never learn that death is permanent. What's the hurry?" (Heilbut, 1984, p. 211)

In 1982, Bettelheim published *Freud and Man's Soul*, which was advanced to be an important reinterpretation of Freudian theory, but which was dismissed by some as yet another example of Bettelheim's "crankiness" (Gay, 1988). Again, the study may be taken both as evidence of his further disillusionment with life in America and as an attempt to clear Freud of the misinterpretations he had suffered at the hands of translators and the language of American psychoanalysis. As Heilbut proposed, despite Bettelheim's former praises of this country's political system, Bettelheim had begun to reveal himself as yet another humanist immigrant horrified by the American intrusion into the territory of his homeland.

When *Freud's Vienna and other Essays* (Bettelheim, 1990) first appeared, reviewers tended to describe it simply as a collection or summary of his beliefs. However, taken as a piece, it seems to more clearly reflect Bettelheim's experience of a nostalgic, painful longing for a return to his cultural roots. It is a reminiscence about the very beginnings of his long intellectual and emotional journey, but also about the loss of an intense emotional tie to Vienna, a Vienna which from his early childhood memories stood as part of a close association "between the city, bread, and water–these basic foods being since most ancient times the symbol of sustenance. To me it was a most convincing association: like my mother, like my home, this larger home in which we all lived, the city, nurtured me well" (Bettelheim, 1990, p. 135).

Trying to make sense of his death, this idea of the loss of the nurturing maternal self-object for Bettelheim, coupled with his sense of stubborn self-righteousness (reflected, for example, in his republishing the long-repudiated article on autistic children, "Feral Children and Autistic Children," in his final essays), brought to mind his early use of the term *messianic* in describing the fantasies of some of the concentration camp prisoners. It thus brought me back to his beginning study, and to the beginning of this paper, which began with a reference to Heinz Kohut's comments on the task of biography.

Kohut's paper is also, interestingly, a study of charismatic and messianic personalities, certain comments in which are reminiscent of Dr. Bettelheim. Kohut describes how when the feelings of security and self-confidence obtained through a merger with powerful self-objects are followed by abrupt and unpredictable frustrations and loss, as certainly happened with Bettelheim in 1939, some premature and overly strenuous attempts at psychological self-restitution appear to bestow on messianic personality types a sense of absolute moral righteousness. This description of the messianic type is consistent with the view presented some years earlier by Arlow and Brenner (1969), who also noted that such illusions may derive from a sense of conflict over guilt-laden aggressive impulses. The sense of righteousness also makes the messianic personality irresistibly attractive to those who need to merge with such self-assured leaders. Thus, during the period of crisis and anxiety associated with World War II and, more specifically, in a time when the field of mental health for children was at a point of just finding its way in the United States, it may have been that there were many who turned to Dr. Bettelheim not simply because of his skills and wisdom, but also because they sensed that he could satisfy their needs to identify with unquestioned righteousness, or with seeming firmness and security.

Unfortunately, as Kohut pointed out, the psychic equilibrium of the messianic leader seems to be an "all-or-nothing" type: there are few survival possibilities between the extremes of utter firmness and strength, on the one hand, and utter destruction, on the other. In line with Kohut's observation, recently published material from personal interviews given by Bettelheim before his death reveals that by 1988, wishes and thoughts about suicide were already on his mind (Fisher, 1990, p. 12). One might speculate that for Bettelheim a growing sense of personal weakness related to an awareness that many of his beliefs were being discredited, the death of his second wife, the progressing infirmities of aging, and the effects of a stroke left him little recourse, in his own mind, but self-destruction or suicide. Further, the accusations about him raised by a few persons in Chicago after his death, and the magnification of those voices by the media, may partly reflect the fact that the idealization of the messianic-like leader, the narcissistic transference to him, can so quickly and easily be thrown aside when the need for it has come to an end.

Bettelheim, the human, is gone, but we have been left with an extensive body of clinical writing, the legacy of an often provocative mind. When all has been said, it will not be forgotten that he was instrumental in promoting a lasting concern about discovering the best treatment methods possible for emotionally disturbed children, and that he successfully fostered a widespread interest for that endeavor in the public at large. He taught many of us, some through direct contact and others through reading, to deeply care and think about the fate of even the most severely impaired children. His arguments, correct or incorrect, continue to stimulate us to unashamedly examine ourselves in our work with troubled youth.

REFERENCES

Aichorn, A. (1935), *Wayward Youth.* New York: Viking.

Arlow, J. A (1959), The structure of the deja vu experience. *J. Amer. Psychoanal. Assn.,* 7:611-631.

Brenner, C. (1969), The psychopathology of the psychosis: A proposed revision. *Internat. J. Psycho-Anal.,* 50:5-14.

Bettelheim, B. (1943), Individual and mass behavior in extreme situations. *J. Abnorm. & Soc. Psychol.,* 38:417-542.

_____ (1947), The concentration camp as a class state. *Mod. Rev.,* 1:628-637.

_____ (1948a), Closed institutions for children. *Bull. Menn. Clin.*, 12:135-142.

_____ (1948b), Somatic symptoms in superego formation. *Amer. J. Orthopsychiat.*, 18:649-658.

_____ (1949), A psychiatric school. *Quart. J. Child Behav.*, 1:86-95.

_____ (1950a), *Love Is Not Enough.* New York: Free Press.

_____ (1950b), Prejudice. *Sci. Amer.*, 186:11-13.

_____ (1952), Schizophrenic art: A case study. *Sci. Amer.*, 186:30-34.

_____ (1955a), Individual autonomy and mass controls. In: Frankfurter *Beitrage zur. Soziologie, vol. 1*, ed. T. W. Adorno & W. Dirks. Aufsatze, Max Horkheimer zum sechzigsten geburtstag gewidment. Frankfurt am Main: Europaische Verlagsanstalt, pp. 245-262.

_____ (1955b), *Truants from Life.* New York: Free Press.

_____ (1956), Schizophrenia as a reaction to extreme situations. *Amer. J. Orthopsychiat.*, 26:507-518.

_____ (1957), Review of *The Life and Work of Sigmund Freud, vol. I* by E. Jones. *Amer J. Sociol.*, 62:418-420.

_____ (1959), Joey: A mechanical boy. *Sci. Amer.*, 200:116-127.

_____ (1960), The ignored lesson of Anne Frank. *Harper's Magazine,* November:45-50.

_____ (1962), Freedom from ghetto thinking. *Midstream,* Spring: 16-23.

_____ (1967a), *The Empty Fortress.* New York: Free Press.

_____ (1967b), Survival of the Jews. (Review of *Treblinka* by J.Steiner.) *New Repub.,* July 1:23-30.

_____ (1969a), Laurie. *Psychology Today,* 2:24-25,60.

_____ (1969b), Obsolete youth: Towards a psychograph of adolescent rebellion. *Encounter,* 33:29-42.

_____ (1972), Youth in turmoil. *Trans. & Stud. Coll. Physicians Phila.*, 39: 179-187.

_____ (1974), *A Home for the Heart.* New York: Alfred A. Knopf.

_____ (1976), *The Uses of Enchantment.* New York: Alfred A. Knopf.

_____ (1982), *Freud and Man's Soul.* New York: Alfred A. Knopf.

_____ (1990), *Freud's Vienna and Other Essays.* New York: A. Knopf.

Janowitz, M. (1949), Ethnic tolerance: A function of social and personal control. *Amer. J. Sociol.*, 55:137-145.

_____ (1950a), *Dynamics of Prejudice.* New York: Harper & Brothers.

_____ (1950b), Reactions to Fascist propaganda—A pilot study. *Pub. Opinion Quart.,* 14:53-60.

_____ Sylvester, E. (1947), Therapeutic influence of the group on the individual. *Amer. J. Orthopsychiat.*, 17 :684-692.

_____ (1948), A therapeutic milieu. *Amer. J. Othopsychiat.*, 18:191-206.

_____ (1949a), Milieu therapy: Indications and illustrations. *Psychoanal. Rev.*, 36:54-68.

_____ (1949b), Physical symptoms in emotionally disturbed children. *The Psychoanalytic Study of the Child*, 314:353-368. New York: International Universities Press.

_____ (1950), Delinquency and morality. *The Psychoanalytic Study of the Child*, 5:329-342. New York: International Universities Press.

Contemporaries: Bruno Bettelheim, Ph.D. (1971), *Mod. Med.*, September 6:18-39,23, 27,31.

Dundes, A. (1991), Bruno Bettelheim's uses of enchantment and abuses of scholarship. *J. Amer. Folklore*, 104:74-83.

Federn, E. (1990), Witnessing psychoanalysis. London: Karnac Books.

Fisher, D. (1990), An interview with Bruno Bettelheim. *LA Psychoanal. Bull.*, Fall:3-23.

Frank, A. (1952), *The Diary of a Young Girl*, trans. B. M. Mooyart–Doubleday. Garden City, NY: Doubleday.

Freud, A. (1963), Regression as a principle in mental development. *Bull. Menn. Clin.*, 27:126-139.

_____ (1965), *Normality and Pathology in Childhood: Assessments of Development.* New York: International Universities Press, 1965.

_____ (1966), *The Ego and the Mechanisms of Defense.* New York: International Universities Press.

Freud, S. (1918), From the history of infantile neurosis. *Collected Papers*, 3:473-607. London: Hogarth Press, 1946.

Gay, P. (1988), *Freud: A Life for Our Time.* New York: W. W. Norton.

Greenacre, P. (1960), Regression and fixation. *J. Amer. Psychoanal. Assn.*,8:703–723.

Heilbut, A. (1984), *Exiled in Paradise.* Boston: Beacon Press.

Henry, J. (1957), Types of institutional structures. *Psychiatry*, 20:47–60.

Horkheimer, M., & Adorno, T. W. (1972), *The Dialectic of Enlightenment*, trans. J. Cumming. New York: Seabury.

Jackson, S.W. (1969), The history of Freud's concepts of regression. *J. Amer. Psychoanal. Assn.*, 17:743-784

Jacobson, E. (1949), Observations on the psychological effect of imprisonment on female political prisoners. In: *Searchlights on Delinquency*, ed. K. R. Eissler. New York: International Universities Press.

_____ (1959), Depersonalization. *Amer. Psychoanal. Assn.*, 7:581-610.

Kohut, H. (1976), Creativeness, charisma, group psychology: Reflections on the self analysis of Freud. In: *The Fusion of Science and Humanism*, ed. J. E. Gedo & G. H. Pollock. *Psychological Issues*, Monograph 34:35. New York: International Universities Press.

Marcovitz, E. (1952), The Meaning of deja vu. *Psychoanal.Quart.*, 21:481-489.

Pucinski, R. (1969), Introduction of Dr. Bettelheim's testimony into the *Congres-*

sional Record–Extentions of Remarks, March 27, 1969, E2473–E2477. Washington, DC: U.S. Govemment Printing Office.

Redl, F. (1942), Group emotion and leadership. *Psychiatry,* 2:573-596.

———— (1943), Group psychological element in discipline problems. *Amer. J. Orthopsychiat.,* 13:77-81.

———— (1944), Diagnostic group work. *Amer. J. Orthopsychiat.,* 14:53-68.

———— (1949), The phenomenon of contagion and "shock effect" in group therapy. In: *Searchlights on Delinquency,* ed. K. R. Eissler. New York: International Universities Press.

———— Wineman, D. (1951), *Children Who Hate.* New York: Free Press.

———— (1952), *Controls from Within: Techniques for the Treatment of the Aggressive Child.* New York: Free Press, 1952.

Sanders, J. (1989), *A Greenhouse for the Mind.* Chicago: University of Chicago Press.

Zimmerman, D. P. (1990), Notes on the history of adolescent inpatient and residential treatment. *Adolescence,* 25:9-38.

———— Sanders, J. (1988), Trends in adolescent inpatient follow–up studies. *Resident. Treat. for Children & Youth,* 6:9-26.

Culture and Residential Treatment

Jacquelyn Sanders, PhD

I wrote this paper when I was asked by a group in Grenoble France to speak about the role of culture in the life of the students at the Orthogenic School. They had invited me to present and explain some aspects of Bettelheim's approach. The very request, of course, is a reflection of the geographical distance of his influence, which extended throughout the world, with his books being published in several languages. The reflection of the profundity of his influence on me is the difficulty that I had when preparing this paper in differentiating among: Bettelheim's ideas, my interpretation of his ideas, my ideas that were influenced by his, and my ideas that might be entirely different from his. I think that this difficulty is not surprising considering all the miles of the merchandise mart that we trod together while looking for just the right furnishings for the Orthogenic School; the many conferences that we had together, with painter, architect, artist, furniture designer; and the many dormitory color selection conferences with students that we mediated together. All of these endeavors were permeated with discussion of both taste and psychology. This is a point of view which I have tried to maintain in our work, to some degree elaborate on, and to teach to others involved in ameliorating lives.

If one considers the meaning of the word "culture," then one might say that it is not *part* of the life of the Orthogenic School, it *is* that life. According to the dictionary, culture refers to careful nurturing and the encouragement of growth. It refers to both the cultivation of humans and the cultivation of plants. Cultivation, this careful encouragement to growth, is at least as important at the beginning of the life of a plant, when the plant is a delicate seedling, as it is at its more mature stages; and perhaps doubly important when the plant is fragile and vulnerable. The same certainly can be said about the beginning of the life of a person and the human states of fragility and vulnerability. Since the task of the Orthogenic School is the careful encouragement to growth of young people who are delicate seedlings, both fragile and vulnerable, culture is essential to its meaning.

Cultivation, of course, needs methods and tools. The arts, literature, dance, painting, sculpture, theater, are some of the tools and methods developed by civilization in the process of humanity's cultivation. In all areas of the work of the Orthogenic School use is made of them. As these tools are used in the education of our young, consideration has to be given as to which are most appropriate to which children and for which purposes. We want our selection to be most helpful in guiding them to mastery of the most important art–the art of living.

A significant aspect of the art of human life is the use of signs and symbols to convey messages. In the arts various modes and senses are used for these signs and symbols. As their use is developed, the more precise are the messages they convey. That is, as language develops we can express ourselves more clearly; and similarly as the skill of painters, sculptors and musicians grow so does the ability to convey complex messages through the arts. Their impact is invariably stronger the more artistically they are conveyed, through modes that will most appropriately touch the receiver. The skill of the political orator influences the public more than a detailed platform treatise, and a declaration of love has greater impact in poetry and song than in a simple statement.

The following discussion of the use of arts at the Orthogenic School will be divided in two. First I will describe and discuss what we do as message givers, and second I will describe and discuss what we do to facilitate our students' ability to become message givers. The basics of what is described were laid down by Bettelheim with embellishment, assistance and variation by generations of staff and students at the Orthogenic School.

The first artistic message that presents itself to the student of the Orthogenic School is the physical structure of the school itself. The exterior is dignified, but not menacing as many institutions can be. The entrance is that part of the School that was originally the minister's home of the adjacent church. The entry door is yellow–it has sometimes been orange–and has always been bright. A graduate once told me of his feeling when he came back to visit. As he approached he could see the yellow door in the distance from across the broad avenue that lies in front of the School. It was like a beacon of warmth across the cold, cold avenue of the world.

On the first visit the child waits for the meeting with the Director, not in a waiting room, but in a living room, furnished for use of children and adults together. There are antiques in the living room–a seahorse from an old carousel, a cradle from Germany, a doll's house, and a bishop's chair–antiques, lovely and delicate, but sturdy enough to be used without excessive care. If you, the reader, can imagine being a small child, anticipating being sent to a strange school because you have been in your life so miserable and perhaps even so bad–you can then imagine the relief you would experience when you walk through a yellow door and past another door that is decorated with colorful figures of angels and fruit–and then into a regular living room that has these old curiosities that you are allowed not only to look at but to touch, play with and even sit on. If you similarly imagine yourself an adolescent or a parent, I am sure that you will agree that this use of artistic productions and artistic arrangement of color and comfort does much more to convey a sense of welcome and warmth than any number of words.

Over the years at the School there has been a considerable amount of building, both new and remodeling. Whenever this was done, the architect became a part of the therapeutic endeavor–and it was his responsibility to understand the messages we wished to convey and to interpret them into the art of architecture. His use of space, for example, was in the service of the interests of the students. Open spaces might be visually satisfying, but our students need limits and clear definitions. The space itself should reflect its purpose. Internally he, therefore, made clear divisions between the living room and eating room–with each having very different textures on wall and floor. Externally he designed a playground that was divided by landscape elements. Rather than have fences to designate different areas, which would have seemed forbidding and restrictive to the children, he had bushes. In our planning sessions he described it as a cross between the Champs Elysee of Paris and the labyrinth of London. In effect we have a very large outdoor area that is lovely looking and clearly divided in a way that seems quite natural. The children can thereby have the idea that controls and limits, like the hedges, can be natural and attractive parts of life rather than unwelcome impositions, like unappealing fences.

In constructing new classrooms the problem was that though all classrooms needed to have similar facilities, in order to combat the ever existing problem of institutionalization, we wanted each to have its own individual character. Of course, each teacher and each class makes that character when they are in the classroom, but we wanted to utilize again the art of architecture to reaffirm this message. Each class, though of similar size, has different flooring (those that are of wood are of different kinds of wood) and different wall covering (one has a shiny wall, one a soft textured wall, and one a straw type matting). They each are colored differently and each conveys a somewhat different feeling.

In the School's buildings there are two enclosed stairhalls. In any institution stairhalls are often the most depressing places. In one of ours there is a ceramic mural whose images go from the bottom of the sea to the top of the mountain. On the way up are various figures of American folklore (Paul Bunyan, the logger, John Henry, the railroader, Pilgrims, Indians, etc.). In the other stairwell there are animals drawn in brightly colored brick. Interesting things transpire in the stairhalls of residential treatment facilities. Not only are there the regular races to see who can get to the top first, or who can jump down the largest number of stairs; but there is also the passing of secret messages, the sitting out of a temper tantrum, or the cooling down of an "I want to be alone" mood. I have, at times, taken a student into a stairhall for a brief but serious conversation, or a scolding that I wanted to do in private, but not in my office. All of these transactions take on a somewhat different tone when watched by characters of culture or wildly beautiful animals, rather than enclosed by shadowy monochromatic walls.

In addition to developing an aesthetic appreciation in those that walk by them, and softening the harshness of an institution, murals like these save money, since they need much less upkeep than painted walls.

These are examples of the art of architecture that supports our therapeutic efforts. We similarly have other works of art in the life of our students. There is an abstract mural on the front of the building, a sculpture of Two Sisters in the courtyard, and on the sides of the drinking fountain in the play yard are graceful bronze figures of children engaged in a variety of physical activities. There are more antiques in the general areas, reproduction of fine art on the walls, and in the dining room and children's living room the chandeliers are of glass and ceramic. These are not just efforts to visually beautify the environment, though that has its merit. All of the art is part of the lives of our young people. By having it close to them, for their intimate use, we let them know how much we value them and how much we trust them. I have been in hospitals where the staff has made very nice efforts to beautify the surroundings, but put the drawings way up high out of the reach of the children. The beauty then is at the same time a constant reminder to these children that they are considered to be inevitably destructive. At a place of residence, things of beauty should be for its residents.

That this message is effective is apparent to any visitor to the Orthogenic School. Though there is the usual amount of slovenliness and disarray in the living areas, that one has to expect of children and adolescents, the School always looks unusually clean and neat for a children's institution. And though there are children who in a temper destroy things, in general the residents do not hurt the furnishings of the school, because they feel that the furnishings are theirs, selected and cared for for them.

Another way that culture is part of the life of the Orthogenic School is in the celebration of holidays around which a variety of traditions have developed. The celebration of holidays in general serves two purposes: that of developing a sense of time, because holidays are significant and obvious time markers in the revolving course of the years; and that of helping children to feel part of a national community. These celebrations can serve an additional purpose in our efforts toward the best "cultivation" of our students. It is our belief that holidays are maintained in the culture of a people because they address basic human needs, and provide a structured and satisfactory way of dealing with some basic human conflicts. We, therefore, organize our celebrations with consideration for those basic human issues that we think the particular holiday symbolizes.

Bettelheim began, and we have continued, a tradition of the school's director talking on the major holidays, with all of the young people together about the significance of the holiday. On Thanksgiving, for example, (which was being celebrated at the time of the writing of this paper) I would let them know that I was sympathetic with the difficulty of this holiday: that given their experience of failure and misery in life they are not likely to be thankful for anything. I would remind them that because of this, usually at the Orthogenic School they were not expected to be thankful for anything. With this reassurance, they could then be reminded that once a year it is appropriate to think of the things for which they can be thankful. It is, after all, important for us all to recognize our good fortune from time to time, and to count our blessings. Such a holiday is a supportive avenue for children to be reminded of this, particularly for children who most of the time should not be expected to be grateful for anything.

The Orthogenic School traditions for this holiday involve eating too much and some reenactment or drawing of the Pilgrims–relating to their successful survival of the winter, and the help they received from the Indians. This theme, of the Pilgrims' successful survival, is a very significant one for children who also come to a new world and have to survive what to them seem to be very great hardships of distressed feelings; and the theme of friendship with natives is very relevant to children who feel themselves to be primitive outcasts, unable to get along with anyone.

Since the students are of various religions, the celebration of Christmas as a religious holiday is optional. However, everyone celebrates the holiday. Its meaningfulness lies in the attitude toward children as being of great value and in the theme of hope in the midst of darkness. The traditions adopted at the Orthogenic School are those most common in the United States, and those adapted from other lands that emphasize these themes. A reflection of the valuableness of children is in their being given thoughtfully selected presents; that of hopefulness, in the bright and lighted Christmas trees. In order for the students to appreciate and receive the message in a beneficial way, there are certain issues that have, invariably to be dealt with. Christmas is always a time of disappointment. In anticipation of the day, the present giving, the family visit, youngsters build up great expectations of having secret desires filled both in terms of presents received and familial love and warmth. The expectations are so high that they must inevitably be disappointed. This, of course, is not an uncommon phenomenon and is particularly intense with severely disturbed youngsters. Such youngsters tend not to be able to be realistic in their expectations and, in addition, tend not be able to have satisfying relationships. When this is openly discussed with them beforehand, it softens the disappointment and they are then more able to appreciate and receive the message of the holiday.

Easter and Passover, the spring holidays, are especially important for our children in the many symbols of hope and new beginnings that are embodied in their traditional celebration. Troubled children need many messages that say they are not alone in having winters of despair, and that such winters do end with springtimes of birth and hope.

The principles that are applied in institutionalized ways to utilizing art and culture to further therapeutic goals are applied in similar fashion in individualized ways about particular issues and with particular children. For example, it is a custom on the anniversary day of a student's coming to the school, to give a present for each anniversary year. Presents are selected to represent something of the student's achievement over the years. In this context we often find art objects to be particularly appropriate–as when a young woman had made great progress in being more accepting of her body, she was given a print of Renoir's bather.

The foregoing has been a discussion of ways of giving messages to young people. The methods and tools of art and culture are also valuable as ways for young people to express themselves and for themselves to give messages. Often there is a back and forth between message givers. For example, we teach our children to read, select works of literature about issues that we think are important for them, and they in turn select literature that tells us what they feel is important for them.

This reciprocity is often reflected in the classroom. When an animal studies unit was presented to a group of preadolescent children, one purpose was to help them deal with some basic primitive issues. Children are attracted to animals because of what they represent in this way–a closeness to their primitiveness. Through discussions of animals they can find out things about themselves. For example, it can be acceptable to talk about bodily processes of animals and their sexual behavior, while talking about such things in relationship to themselves might make some children too anxious. As part of this class, in addition to the lessons prepared and presented by their teacher, each student chose an animal as an independent study project. The animals they chose invariably represented characteristics of themselves. The study of the animal was helpful then in the expression of and to some extent coming to terms with that characteristic. The most aggressive boy, for example, chose sharks; a boy concerned about his own intelligence chose the dolphin.

A group of adolescents, who were very difficult to engage in most academics, found the study of Indian tribes quite fascinating. Discussion of their rituals and practices, their culture, relates to many issues with which our young people contend. In a discussion for example, of the hallucinogenic effect that some of the initiation practices have, the issues that lead present day youth to seek such experiences could be aired in a non-threatening way. Use of culture need not be only of our own culture. There is much to be learned from the practices of other cultures and of more primitive cultures. Since the practices are different, less taken for granted, it is sometimes easier to see and understand the issues that lie behind them. The initiation rites of a primitive culture are often clearly designed to help the adolescent feel capable of entering adult life. It is easier then to see and, therefore, discuss the issue of every adolescent's insecurity in entering adulthood.

In such a class the questions that the students raise, the practices that they find most peculiar, are often closely related to important issues in themselves. For example, one boy thought it was very outrageous that a particular Indian tribe did not know or pronounce the name of their god. This was an interesting comment since the boy's family was of the Orthodox Jewish faith and also were forbidden to pronounce the name of their god. Furthermore, the boy was adopted and did not know a very significant name–that of his biological parents.

Television and comic books are a significant part of popular art and culture. They can be viewed as the fairy tales of our time. Like fairy tales, their popularity is very much dependent on their appeal to very basic human interests; unlike fairy tales they have not yet passed the test of time. At the Orthogenic School what students watch on television, at the movies or the theater, and what they read, are considered to be significant parts of their environment. Because of this we are very careful in their selection and pay attention to the choices made.

The amount and selection of television programs are limited more than the amount and selection of reading material. Reading is a more active process than watching television. Furthermore, the emotions aroused while reading a book are more easily integrated than those aroused while watching television. If a disturbing scene is shown on television, one does not have time to cope with it before another scene is shown. Whereas when reading a book one can stop and reflect, can put the book down and go back to it another time. Students are, therefore, not allowed to watch one program immediately after another. The programs that they watch are preselected and they watch one program at a time so that it is possible to reflect on, discuss, and digest what is stimulated. When handled in this way, the values of good television are much the same as the values of good theater and good literature. That is, they can give to the child important messages, convey important values, and offer solutions to important conflicts. At the same time, the selection made by the child of particular programs can tell us a great deal of the interests and concerns of that child.

Since disturbed youngsters in general have great difficulty in dealing with their aggressiveness, we tend to avoid the stimulation of violent feelings. In our experience the effect or value the depiction of violence has, however, seems to be an individual matter, depending both on how the issue of violence is presented and resolved, and on the psychological stage of development of the individual watching or reading about the violence. When, for example, one of our boys was fascinated with violence, we suggested that he read Remarque's *All Quiet on the Western Front,* a very graphic but sensitive portrayal of the senseless violence of war. This book was a more effective and convincing argument against war than anything we ever said.

When another boy was fascinated with violent books and expressed interest in seeing violent movies, we limited his doing so, but paid attention to his reactions and discussed the books with him. It became clear that, in limited quantities, he was neither overstimulated nor made anxious by the reading of the books or watching of the movies. This interest, in fact, seemed in keeping with his growing maturity and commitment to law and order. We had no record of this boy's early history. According to his adoptive parents, there was reason to believe that there was physical trauma in his early years. We, therefore, speculated that reading and seeing violence was a way to help him master some unconscious memories.

Some popular comic books seem to serve some functions similar to those served by fairy tales; that is, for instance, as morality tales. Superman is not as old as Jack the Giant Killer, but the story of the shy young man's ability to turn stronger than any villain has some of the same components as Jack's story. There are now many other super heroes; though some are anti-heroes, many are clear heroes whose stories always guarantee the victory of right over wrong. They also incorporate some of the advances of modern technology and, thereby, become more appropriate fairy tales of the times.

The uses that children make of these comics vary. We have had at times a boy who would retreat into the comic books and, to some extent, this would be a substitution for life. It has been more usual, however, that if we show respect for their interest, and express interest in it, the comic books become an avenue for communication. It seems consistent that most youngsters who are fascinated by the super hero comics, gain some feeling of security from the fantasy that the weak, the malformed, the strange, can become strong in some magical way and overcome evil forces that are aligned against them. The particulars of the fascination vary from child to child, depending a great deal on the child's self-perception. Because of this identification, our expressed interest in the comic book super hero can be experienced as interest in the child.

In work with children who are limited in their ability to communicate and terrified of revealing themselves, to view such interests as selection of books, television programs, and comic books as communication is vitally important. When we can indicate by our response that their interests and desires are acceptable and understandable, they become more ready to communicate in other ways as well.

Because of our students' limitations or inhibitions in the more ordinary modes of communication, the expressive arts are especially important; not as a means for so-called free expression, but as a means for the development of expressive and communicative ability.

The development of movement has deeper value, also. Our youngsters are all beset with bodily anxieties, frequently afraid to move. It is, therefore, an important part of our program to help them develop comfort with their bodies and the feeling of mastery. This can often be enhanced by teaching athletic and movement skills. To teach these well requires sensitivity to the children so that the teaching can begin at the level of the child, with appropriate understanding and consideration for the extreme anxiety that accompanies movement. Since our children need a great deal of help in being able to manage competitive feelings, and since they are usually terrified of failure, we have to be very careful in monitoring competition in sports activities, and de-emphasizing the performance aspect of movement skills. Since the first ego is the body ego, the improved sense of self that comes of bodily mastery is always evident with such physical accomplishment.

We teach the plastic arts as another form of expression with somewhat different rules. They provide another avenue that can be directly related to an individual's uniqueness. It can sometimes be a mode wherein the person is more effective than in other modes. However, just as it is necessary to master language in order to express oneself adequately and communicate verbally; and just as it is necessary to master one's bodily movements in order to dance in a satisfying and attractive way; so is it necessary to master the modes and tools of plastic expression in order to express oneself adequately and communicate effectively in an artistic way.

In my experience we have had a number of moderately and two truly talented artists in residence at the Orthogenic School. The one was unable to paint when her inner forces were too disruptive. If she tried, her paintings were too chaotic. The other was able to use her skills throughout the course of her treatment. It was very evident that she utilized these skills in the service of maintaining her integration. For many years the expression of her creativity was in form rather than in content. She would, for example, make intricate and elaborate quilts of pleasing design and color. It was only toward the end of her treatment that she began to have content in her productions. It seems that if she had attempted such an expression earlier, the chaos for her, too, would have disrupted her skills. When she had greater emotional strength, she could couple her imagination with her talent and produce remarkably beautiful images. One of the last works that she did at the Orthogenic School could be interpreted as a moving message. It was a quilt of fantastic animals designed by her–a message that warmth, imagination and skill can all be integrated to enhance life.

In this review of the use of culture at the Sonia Shankman Orthogenic School, I have tried to exemplify how art and culture can be used to convey messages to children; how children can use the art and culture of others to convey their own personal messages; and how they can gradually, at times, learn to create their own art that conveys, in turn, universal messages.

The Child Care Worker
and the Youth with Character Disorder

Joseph D. Noshpitz, MD

SUMMARY. This presentation is designed to address the management issues posed by youngsters in residence with serious symptoms of character disorder. The introductory material reviews some of the more salient behaviors associated with this syndrome, and the general measures invoked to deal with the condition. The bulk of the paper addresses the issue of how the child care worker can most usefully respond to these behaviors, and a three level style of response is described. These levels consist of First Tier: Reflecting the behavior in an empathic fashion; Second Tier: Relating the behavior to some underlying wish or fantasy; Third Tier: interpreting the unconscious roots of the defensive character of this wish/behavior pattern. Illustrations are offered as to how these levels are actually translated into teachable responses.

Despite all the to do about least restrictive environment, inappropriate hospitalization and mounting costs of mental health care, the gritty reality which faces all sizable communities and all too many families is the impact of the many adolescents who need inpatient placement. One of the typical responses our society makes to this has been to offer these youngsters short term care. The result was predictable; within a given year, a troubled youth may go through three placements, one for thirty days, one for forty five days, and one for ten days, passing back and forth among several settings as each effort either runs out of funding or refuses further to put up with the difficulties this troublesome patient poses. The extravagant wastefulness of such an approach is exceeded only by its therapeutic ineffectiveness. Indeed, if anything, it is countertherapeutic, since it subjects the patient successively to one group of interveners after another, each of whom seeks to build a relationship and develop a modicum of trust and closeness, and each of whom in turn interrupts, detaches and withdraws its relationship bid. With what effects on its clients can all too easily be imagined.

With even cursory study it is evident that the youngsters who are going through this are for the most part representatives of that great class of psychiatric categories today called personality disorders. The symptomatology of this group of conditions is not clear enough to be considered a primary psychiatric illness–it does not get them listed as Axis I in the official nomenclature. Yet the evident seriousness of their symptoms is of such proportions as to create a veritable crisis in care with many profound social overtones. All the ambiguities of our societal values are here–these conditions overflow into the group assigned to the penal system and its practitioners, into the ranks of the learning disabilities addressed by special educators, into the coterie cared for by those who deal with victims of drug and alcohol abuse, and, in many instances, into a common borderland with the mentally retarded. Thus, within the professional world, the provinces of many hands and the processes of many different service systems may be the points of entry into care. Ultimately, however, the more seriously disturbed among these youngsters, whether identified in juvenile court, in special ed class at school, or wherever, tend to be referred to some facet of the mental health system. And the matter of their needs and their management must be addressed in that context.

As noted, after outpatient efforts have failed, the acute, short term unit sees them first, officially for evaluation. A characteristic recommendation that arises from such a study is for long term care. All too often, however, such long term care does not exist or is not immediately available; many are the horror stories of youngsters waiting for months or years, or being sent out of state to where the treatment agency cannot be supervised, the parents cannot visit very easily, and many unfortunate complications then ensue. Depending on the locality or funding source, all sorts of arbitrary decisions are made: such children can be placed only in long term hospitals; such children can be placed only in non-hospital residential treatment centers, or only in intermediary care facilities with an upper limit of nine months stay, etc.

Meanwhile, whatever its nature, the setting that *would* undertake the care for such youngsters is faced with a formidable challenge. What exactly is a personality disorder and how does one treat it?

There are various formulations about the nature of personality. Gunderson (1989, p. 2634) speaks of the historical shift from the earlier intrapsychic approach which viewed personality structures as compromises and defenses organized around psychic conflict, to the more current interpersonal approach which defines personality as "the person's characteristic pattern of participation in activities with the world." There was a corresponding shift from defense analysis to such social therapies as community and family models. As this transformation was taking place, several recent streams of therapeutic effort cut new furrows in the fallow fields of treatment potential. The work of Kohut (1971), Kernberg (1984), and the self-psychologists (Ornstein, A. 1981) opened up novel channels of possibility for individual therapy. Moreover, the studies of Marohn (1980), Masterson (1972), Rinsley (1980), and others began to expand these ideas and apply them to inpatient care.

To return to explorations into the nature of personality, however, Millon (1981) speaks of "ingrained and habitual ways of psychological functioning that emerge from the individual's entire developmental history, and which, over time, come to characterize the child's "style." In sum, a "personally distinctive style of coping with others and relating to ourselves. . . " (p. 8) " . . .a complex pattern of deeply embedded psychological characteristics that are largely unconscious, cannot be eradicated easily, and express themselves automatically in almost every facet of functioning–the individual's distinctive pattern of perceiving, feeling, thinking and coping."

Whatever definition one employs, it is likely to convey a sense that the disorder is first, pervasive, that is to say, that it is expressed in every aspect of the individual's life; second, that it is enduring, and will be found in one form or another as a consistent presence over time. And third, that it enjoys the favor of the individual, who perceives this mode of getting along as "myself," "my personal style," "my way of thinking, and feeling, and doing things." The individual may be unhappy with this style, the shyness or aggressiveness, the impulsiveness or moodiness, but, paradoxically, is likely to resist efforts to change it–any intimations to change these characteristics are experienced as implicit criticisms or outright threats, or even as frank invasions of the self. Often enough the person with such a condition is driven to seek help only when life has become intolerable, and the negative consequences of these preferred adaptive modes finally come to outweigh the investment in maintaining them. For the most part, with all the difficulties up to that point, the individual had nonetheless arrived at a personal equilibrium, a deeply ingrained, well practiced mode of living, the product of a lifetime of effort. There is an implicit statement to the world: You'll have to take me as I am. Thus, in the nature of things, this person cannot readily welcome an offer to help change. At that point the familiar distinction between what is ego-syntonic and what ego-dystonic becomes both very real and very substantial.

The personality disorder diagnoses which bring youngsters into consideration for long term care are usually distributed among the psychopathic, the borderline, the narcissistic, the schizotypal, and the paranoid. (Perhaps the commonest formulation is: Personality Disorder, Mixed Type with Narcissistic and Impulsive Features.) Other personality disorder categories such as dependent, avoidant, compulsive, passive-aggressive, and histrionic are usually accompanied by less severe symptoms and do not invite so intensive an approach. In any case, the key criterion is the element of intolerable behavior involving family members, the school, the community, or directly affecting the patient himself.

The management of such youngsters then becomes a matter of defining the relevant areas of pathology, and designing appropriate strategies to undertake the necessary repairs. There are several symptom clusters that must be addressed. To begin with, there is the chronic instability in the basic adaptive makeup of many of these individuals; they react to stress in idiosyncratic and excessive ways which are calculated to disrupt the composure of others in their immediate vicinity. There is their difficulty in the regulation of affect. They speak of being depressed, of thinking constantly about revenge, of being angry much of the time, or perhaps, most commonly of all, of sudden, radical, inexplicable mood shifts. To counter these noxious emotions, they seek some external means for attempting to reestablish a sense of well-being. Often enough, this carries them into the outer reaches of pathology. Thus, temper outbursts, smoking, alcohol or other substance abuse, promiscuity, or skin cutting might all be means toward this end. The characteristic forms of ego and superego pathology are often in evidence, with lying, manipulating, stealing, dissimulating, keeping hidden caches of contraband about, plotting various illicit maneuvers, and otherwise maintaining a covert behavioral pattern parallel with what they allow the staff to see. This might be complemented by explosive outbursts of violence, threats (to staff and patients alike), negativistic and defiant behavior, deliberate and exhibitionistic violations of rules, sexual deviance, and a host of similar challenges, provocations, and power struggles.

Confronting these clusters of symptoms and behavior is the everyday work of the treatment team, and, in particular, of the child care staff. Their daily problem is: How to deal with the behavior–what to say, what to do?

The pathology exists on many levels. There are ego deficits, superego problems, interpersonal distortions, delinquent value systems, odd social affiliations (devil worship, cults, gangs, etc.), and intricate forms of family pathology–all of which have to be addressed. The therapeutic systems which have evolved have borrowed from many disciplines. The average treatment setting includes a wide variety of tactics modeled upon behavioral psychology and using some form of operant conditioning to shape behavior. This has led to reward systems involving tokens, points, or privileges, a graduated hierarchy of levels to be attained by conforming behavior, time out, room time, and quiet room containment. Hospital practice has contributed experience with various shades of partial or total seclusion, and restraints. Psychopharmacology offers tantalizing but unpredictable possibilities of alleviating depression, stopping impulsive and explosive outbursts, relieving anxiety, reversing psychotic regression, and calming the hyperactive attention of the ADHD youngster. (Like everything else we try, sometimes it works, and sometimes it doesn't.) Educational tactics abound to cope with the omnipresent cognitive deficiencies which burden these youngsters.

Individual psychotherapy seeks to get directly at the underlying dynamics. Family therapy in all its varieties tries to come to grips with the often shattered and scattered familial fragments which had in large measure engendered the patient's pathology, and which often enough now seek to perpetuate it. An array of community meetings is likely to be in place to give patients a sense of the meaning of their lives and behavior in relationship to others. Group therapy further accentuates the role of interpersonal significance as the setting for the individual life, and offers buffer and model for the expression of inner turmoil. An educational apparatus is present to foster the growth and enrichment of the youngster's cognitive capacities, and a series of specialized expressive therapies to channel and give tongue to non-verbal affective promptings. All of these are by now routinely built into the large majority of settings, but withal, they are effective only to the extent that they are matched by special individualized routines of relationship and companionship which are offered to each youngster by the child care staff.

Given such a number and variety of instruments of intervention, there is an evident need for some way of orchestrating this diverse group. It is here that the contributions of dynamic psychiatry and psychoanalysis begin to fulfill their promise. In my view, these approaches remain the most useful bodies of theory we have available in terms of understanding why patients act as they do. Certainly these theories offer a greater possibility of making sense out of the chaotic behavior the staff encounters than do any other approaches. Nonetheless, they remain the most difficult to integrate into milieu practice. Applying psychodynamic constructs involves a considerable leap from a framework of theory and schema of meaning to the immediacies of behavior. That has proven extraordinarily difficult to translate into milieu practice. The formulations of psychoanalysis were designed for use with patients whose supine position required a complete containment of any action–except free association and verbalization. This realm of the verbal and the expressive was based a priori on the inhibition of action. Indeed, when the patient reported behavior which took place away from the session but with the suggestion that it was an expression of tensions arising from within the analytic situation, such behavior was labeled as acting-out. The patient was asked forthwith to stop doing that and to analyze these tensions instead.

How then to apply principles arising from such a system to a milieu whose very nature is action. In the milieu context, much of what transpires is communication via enactment–the enactment of conscious and unconscious conflicts, the direct expression of lust and rage, the oblique and covert embodiment of pathological character structures in sly, devious, and manipulative behavior–and so on and on for a host of non-verbal or pseudoverbal devices.

Over the years, there have been a number of important efforts to make this translation, and some gifted authors have undertaken the burden of bridging these realms. Such outstanding figures as August Alchhorn, Bruno Bettelheim, and Fritz Redl come immediately to mind as the classic figures in the field. Additional contributions have come from Stanislaus Zurich, Fritz Meyer, and others. More recently, the work of Donald Holmes, Donald Rinsley, and Richard Marohn have enriched the approaches to this effort. Withal however, no single teachable system has emerged to offer a universally accepted constructive methodology for the work of the child care staff. Such a design will probably be the outcome of a slow accumulation of concepts and practices. With the passage of time, these will gradually diffuse among the practitioners of this discipline, and will grow by accretion as more and more efforts are undertaken to explore the details of the terrain whose larger dimensions our predecessors have mapped for us. The following suggestions are offered as one small and tentative step in that long trek which lies ahead.

There are many kinds of interventions which child care staff are required to make. They are meeting both the developmental needs of their young charges, and the therapeutic requirements stirred by the youngsters' syndromes. At different moments, staff members are mother, father, sibling, therapist, friend, mentor, counselor, grandparent, parent trainer, Dutch uncle, jailer, teacher, and executioner–depending on the context. We cannot discuss all these dimensions of relationship, and we cull out of these many roles the specific subgroup of situations which require the counselor/therapist input. The child care worker is usually not the primary therapist (except, perhaps, in Bettelheim's setting), but is typically an important auxiliary therapist. This role is crucial, for the characteriological stuff we face is not lightly altered. It is tough and durable; patterns of stealing, manipulating, substance abuse, violence, crudeness, obscenity, impulsive lashing out–these are curiously tenacious traits and do not give way readily to our therapeutic approaches. Whether we work supportively, suppressively, or interpretively, it is likely to be slow going, with changes coming only gradually and episodically, and many weeks and months of enduring the youngster's affronts lying in store.

It is for that reason in particular that we need a containing setting and an expert staff. For to carry out such treatment, the efforts of each individual child care worker are crucial. Indeed, to the extent that we attempt to perform the specific task of working with character structures, the contribution of the child care staff is an essential component of the therapeutic action. To deal with personality problems, one aspect of the treatment effort is the veritable erosion of these stubborn, egosyntonic character defenses—with the interpretive efforts of the various staff members acting as do wind and water when they play against the refractory substance of the mountain. There has to be a repetitive convergence of the various individual efforts, with each one bearing an analogous message, to achieve the erosive/confrontative effort we are after.

In practice, we cannot address these characteriologic issues without developing a considerable level of trust between youngster and caretakers. To do this, the patients must first experience the staff as offering them both structure and empathy. Trust requires both. Predictability and a respect for principles must be wedded to a sensitivity for each youngster's plight and a sense of compassionate resonance with that youngster's pain. A tall order, that, and a goal toward which to strive rather than a given with which to begin. But in terms of technique, we can try to sharpen the efforts of the child care worker by offering a set of things to say, a way of undertaking this set of tasks and carrying it through.

Toward this end, we have to begin by recognizing what form of empathic support a given youngster requires and finding ways to extend it. With the help of Kohut's approach, we can begin to teach the child care worker how to be a good mirror, the kind of mirror a given youth needs at a critical moment. The theory behind this effort is simple: the various acting out syndromes are seen as deficiency diseases. During early childhood a vital ingredient had been omitted, and the patient's current behavior—and self-organization—is a consequence of this essential deprivation. The missing element is adequate caretaker empathy; the treatment is the provision of adequate replacement therapy. What the child care worker says, the specific empathic reflections, have to be carefully orchestrated so that they mesh both with the planful structure of the program in general and with the specific interpersonal context in which they are offered. They will often have to be part of limit setting, e.g., when a certain amount of grandiose manipulation has earned a narcissistic youngster some loss of privilege, it might be communicated in such terms as "I know how important it is to feel in control of things, how uncomfortable it can make a person to feel that someone else is running the show. But the rules are the rules and everyone has to follow them, etc." Thus, the impersonality of law is pitted against the specific need of a particular youth–the need is recognized and acknowledged, even as the law is also enforced.

In fact, the technique of reflection is only a first step on the level of understanding. What I am suggesting here is a three tier approach, with empathic mirroring as the first working level. There are then second and third steps to follow. This first step, structure and empathy, is designed to build trust. The second step is embarked on after a measure of relationship and trust has been established. In terms of what the child care worker says it sounds much like the first level, except that now one adds an additional increment of understanding, one speaks to the conscious but not usually verbalized wish behind the action. The youngster who tries to control everything that goes on does not merely seek control; behind this behavior may be a variety of yearnings, e.g., the wish to be seen as the important and commanding figure in the group, or the wish to be admired for being so smart and able and strong and calling the shots, or the wish to protect oneself from any possible threat from any quarter (if one is in control, one can't be messed with), etc. The treatment team meets and talks about what the youngster is ready to hear, and, when the time is adjudged to be right, the various exchanges with child care staff now begin to include some reference to the conscious but unexpressed underlying wish. The hoped for effect of such comments is to make this behavior discussable, to begin to weaken the hold of this method of dealing with problems on the youngster's coping style.

Finally, the third tier of comments are more directly connected to motivations that are unconscious, or incompletely conscious. Thus, one might say: "I wonder sometimes if you don't have to be such a big shot all the time because way down underneath you feel so small and helpless and vulnerable, and you try to hide that both from yourself and from other people by acting like you are king of the hill." Or, one might talk to a macho young man about his feeling of lack of manliness, or his yearning to be a baby and be taken care of–whatever it seems is the most accessible dimension of the youngster's adjustment difficulties.

There is a special kind of problem inherent in the psychodynamic approach which must be addressed at the outset. It has to do with the way the human mind reaches a decision. Almost any position we take, any action we initiate, any conclusion we reach, is almost invariably the outcome of a multitude of motivational vectors simultaneously at work. In other words, we do not do things for a reason; we do them for a multitude of reasons, some urging toward that course of action, some inclining us to an alternative channel of expression, and some seeking to wave us off and avoid the issue entirely. It is the summation of this host of motivational factors that finally determines what we do–or do not do. The defining characteristic of dynamic theory lies precisely in this recognition of the multi-determination of decision/action/behavior. And it is in tracing out and exploring the many many roots of a given wish or act that such a theoretical approach finds its richest realization. (This stands in marked contrast to behavioral theory, where ever greater specificity of a single stimulus or operant is looked to as the specific determinant of behavior.)

In the nature of things, however, this very multi-determination of behavior also confronts a treatment team with a formidable obstacle. Given the fact that a host of perhaps widely different motivations lie behind a given act, how does one know which one of these to talk to? Which of the many possible determinants does one address?

Let us look at a concrete example. A common problem on many inpatient units for adolescents is the presence of youngsters who cut, burn, or tattoo their skin in a variety of ways. This has many forms and degrees, and it is related to a variety of self-injurious acts such as hand scraping, banging one's fists or knuckles against a wall, banging one's head against some hard object, and the like. Like all such masochistic patterns, this behavior has a remarkably lengthy and complex list of determinants. Understanding and coping with this array of behaviors is of particular importance to clinicians because these comprise, or are associated with, the single greatest class of resistances to improvement. It is one of the great paradoxes of modern psychiatric medicine that some of the sickest and neediest patients fight treatment with all the energy they can muster; the self-destructive coterie is the most tenaciously resistant of them all. Hence it is especially important to strive to understand the multiple meaning of their behavior. What follows then is an attempt to give some indication of what the more commonly encountered motives of such behavior might be. As we will see, even a partial listing of these underlying mechanisms (we can never assemble more than a partial listing–the behavior simply has too many determinants to allow for anything like a complete exploration) opens the door to a wide range of potential interventions:

1. The youngster feels guilty about some real or fancied wrongdoing and is seeking self-punishment–or at any rate expiation–to pay for the wrongdoing by the skin cutting or burning. Unlike most instances of skin cutting, this particular motive can lead to suicidal behavior.

2. Allied to that might be the feeling of such fear of the potential retaliation–or such a need to control what happens–that the youngster prefers to do the punishing before others can inflict it. This is often associated with other megalomania fantasies; underlying the behavior is a more or less covert sense of omnipotence, a fantasy of dominating of the environment.

3. The act may be in the service of defiance. One demonstrates one's autonomy by violating the rules. No one can make you stop hurting yourself–that's something *you* decide. By hurting yourself when "they" don't want you to, you emerge the victor, you "win" the power struggle.

4. In contrast to this, a youngster may feel suicidal but be afraid to say so. Or perhaps there is a terrifying sense of imminent loss of control. The self-injurious behavior then is in fact an alerting mechanism, a cry for help, a signal of one's desperation.

5. Some youngsters, particularly those who have been abused,

have learned early on that any closeness or intimacy with their caretaker was inevitably associated with pain. Curious admixtures of pleasure and pain ensue, so that ultimately a system is set up where injury and/or pain are linked to erotic excitement. It is around such a nidus that a sadomasochistic perversion forms; directed against the self, the skin cutting is then a form of masturbation.

6. Sometimes this kind of behavior gets caught up in a compulsive ritual. One performs compulsive acts in general in order to relieve anxiety. The skin cutting may subserve such a function and be resorted to compulsively whenever anxiety is aroused. Under such circumstances, there is an intense sense of relief once the act is performed.

7. This behavior may be driven by interpersonal needs. Thus, one uses it as a kind of blackmail: look what you're making me do, I do this because of the way you treat me. In effect, the powerful lever of suffering at someone is leaned on by this enactment.

8. The interpersonal dimension can also involve attention seeking. Deprived children in particular, with their enormous unsatisfied hunger for maternal connectedness, will speak of, and act on, their need for adult responsiveness–they call it a need for attention. They yearn to be noticed, to be the center of attention, and self-injury is a dependable means of grabbing for this prize.

9. In some individuals, the primary yearning is for display. They have erotized attention and get a thrill out of exhibiting. It is reassuring to see the shock and concern that will greet the display of their damage; they get quite a reward from the impact they make.

It is evident that in dealing with the skin cutter, the richness of themes to be considered, only a few of which are listed above, makes for a considerable challenge to a therapeutic team. Any of the above motivations might be at work, or, more typically still, several of them are present at once and come together to urge the youngster into action. Clearly, there has to be some way to integrate the activity of the various team members so as to address one particular facet of this array, the one most strategically available for work at that juncture. Hence team meetings and clinical decision work are always necessary.

There is another point that must be made about such "talking therapy." The fact is that, generally speaking, no one comment, empathic or interpretative, can bring about the necessary changes. These are characteriologic structures we are seeking to change; they have resilience, durability, and, through long habituation, a readiness to be evoked automatically in the face of stress. They are like fixed, rigid beliefs which are clung to as though they were handholds on a sheer cliff; they are survival mechanisms and they will not be given up easily. More to the point, they are systems of meanings, at once disturbed and treasured, and we need to address them with an array of alternative and corrective meanings. Hence, it takes many many repetitions of appropriately phrased comments to begin to impinge on such ego structures in any effective way, and it has to come from people whom the patient has come to trust, and who form the human backdrop to the youth's current experience.

To illustrate these points in greater detail, let me offer a few such three tier formulations which can be employed by child care staff. For the moment let us continue with the theme of the skin cutting we have embarked on. It is important to recognize that in general, such behavior is often associated with some magical fantasy, with the sense of the self as omnipotent, as controlling one's world through the self-injurious act. Given so rich and various an array of determinants, it is evident that no single formulation can address all these issues at once. Nor is it appropriate to do so. Sooner or later the issues must indeed be addressed, but the order in which this is carried out will vary widely from case to case. In any given individual, certain aspects of the underlying matrix of causes will be closer to the surface than others; the key to management is to sort out which one is now most approachable and to concentrate on that. For example, a youngster acts up, gets some sort of restriction, and within minutes is bleeding from three long parallel scratches on his arm. As the staff discusses what is happening, many aspects and possible meanings of the behavior are reviewed, and presently a particular formulation is arrived at.

> First Tier: I guess you're telling us how you felt about the restriction.
> Second Tier: I think that when you get restricted you feel you're losing control of the situation. So you do this, and now, you're back in charge. You are making this happen, it is not the

staff who calls the turn with our restrictions, it is you with your cutting. What a feeling of power that gives you–it makes you feel like the boss of what happens.

There's another side to it as well. I think you are trying to set up a system of blackmail: if you teach us that restricting you leads to this kind of self-damage, maybe you can scare us off, train us to be afraid of restricting you because look what happens.

Third Tier: When you were little, you felt small, and hurt and wounded and helpless. Now you're trying to turn the tables on those feelings by making yourself into the guy who controls everything. Even if it has to be by hurting yourself; it is better to be the one in charge, than to be back to where you were as a little child, where other people did the hurting, and you were their victim.

Now let us change the situation and look at some other kinds of problem behaviors. Let us assume that a youngster has been involved in some fairly serious deception and has had some disciplinary action meted out to her. In discussing it later with a child care worker, initially the worker might say something like:

I guess it was important for you to show us what a good liar you are, how slick you are, how slick you are at covering up, how well you can pull the wool over everybody's eyes, how innocent you can act when you've got all sorts of hot items tucked out of sight. It's impressive, you're really a master at it.

One can press the theme further, e.g., Where did you learn to do that, did someone teach it to you or did you figure it out without any coaching or guidance?

At the second tier level the comment might be: I guess you like to be in control of all the situations in your life–and the best way you've found to do that is to keep everyone guessing. You know what's going on and they don't–so you're in control of what's happening, and they're all blundering around in the dark. That's real power.

Third Tier: Sometimes a gal has been through a lot of situations where she has felt helpless. She was abused, she was neglected, she was exploited–and she was in the hands of grownups who didn't care, and who used her for their purposes. So she learned that by covering up and putting on an act, she could seem to please this one and satisfy that one, and meanwhile, behind the scenes, she was getting some of what she wanted. But she could never get enough, never get what she really needed, and she was never ever able to feel sure of herself. Sometimes she wondered whether she had brought it all on herself; whether she really deserved for things to be any better. If people knew the truth about her, it would be awful. So, in order to feel safe, she had to keep on doing it, more and more of it. After all, it was the best that she could do, and it has always felt safer to put on an act, to lie, to cover up; that way she could have some control of her life, and at the same time, keep people from knowing what a bad person she is.

Let us take another example. Let us assume that the character trait with which we are seeking to come to grips is a constant pattern of accusation. One of the commonest ones the child care worker is likely to encounter goes something like this: I'm perfectly OK. The only problem I have is being locked up and having to stay in here. You're my trouble, you're the ones who are messing me up. If it weren't for you I'd get along fine.

First tier: That's pretty smart. When you come at people like that, it keeps them off balance, makes everybody else wonder if they are guilty, makes everybody else defend themselves. That way, it's not your problem, you're doing all right. It's their problem, they're the ones who are misbehaving. Pretty neat, pretty slick. (In short, what one reflects is the youngster's skill at manipulative verbal acrobatics.)

Second tier: In a way, it makes very good sense to keep accusing other people, makes a person feel in the right; you are not to blame for anything, you are a victim. You don't have a problem; you are the one who is being mistreated or dealt with unfairly. They should be apologizing to you for the bad things they have done to you. (Thus, one speaks to the wish to avoid looking at one's own problem, and the use of projection to accomplish this.)

Third tier: I get a feeling that somewhere inside you you

blame yourself for whatever happens. Like there's some inner voice in you that keeps accusing you of doing bad things or thinking bad thoughts. And that is so painful that to get some relief, you turn that out on other people and accuse them. In a way, it's a better feeling to be the accuser than to feel that the finger is always pointing at you–but inside, that's what you feel.

We have already considered a situation where grandiose manipulation was the issue. To review that within our present framework, the management might go like this.

First Tier: You're telling us that you're the top man, you are the best there is, you are smarter, slicker, quicker, slier, trickier, more clever than anyone around. You're lots smarter than the staff, you can run rings around them, outwit them every time. Must be a great feeling. You may get caught sometimes, but there are so many times that you get away with it and don't get caught, that the few times you do slip up hardly matter. In fact, that proves how great you are–that you get caught so seldom. (One can then go on to invite the youngster to tell of his exploits: what do you think your best trick was?)

Second Tier: One of the good things about being the greatest is that once he gets there, a guy never has to worry. He never has to think about someone else getting everybody's attention or interest–after all, people will be thinking about and noticing the best (or the bravest, the smartest, the toughest, etc.).

Third Tier: Somewhere inside you seem to feel that you haven't got what it takes, that no one will notice you or care for you or pay you any attention, that in yourself, you're not worth their caring about. Only if you can become the greatest and most important can you get away from that awful inside feeling of not being worth anything or of not deserving anything.

Where the problem is one of invasive defiant provocativeness:

First Tier: It seems real important to you to make people angry with you. You go way out of your way to say or do things that get them all upset with you and mad at you.

Second Tier: Maybe there's something you are after that you

can get only by getting people mad at you. I think you get a certain relief that way, you feel more relaxed when that happens. It's actually more comfortable and feels safer to be on the outs with everyone, than to take a chance on being friendly–because that's when a guy can be hurt, or let down, or disappointed.

Third Tier: I think there's a part of you inside that hates you, and that keeps telling you to destroy yourself or to act in a way that will make other people want to destroy you. It's like trying to escape from inside punishment by making the world into an outside punisher. As long as you can keep the outside world attacking you, you're paying your dues. You don't have to pay attention to that inner punisher; for the time being he'll let you be. But you can't stop; the minute you quit provoking people, you begin to feel that nagging inner voice telling you how bad you are. That builds up a kind of pressure inside, and that's why you feel so relieved when you are punished.

Where the issue is a girl's sexual provocativeness, our usual way of delivering a reproof or demanding an alteration in behavior is to call her behavior "inappropriate" or "unacceptable." This generally refers to the shame dimension of the behavior; the specific activity is often never mentioned as such. In effect, we are condemning the behavior by inference and innuendo. It is probably better to speak directly and explicitly, thus:

First Tier: It seems to mean a lot to you to realize that by dressing in this way or acting like that you can get males sexually excited. You keep presenting yourself in a way that says: Look at me, I'm sexually interesting, look at my bosom, look at my crotch, I'm exciting, I'm available.

Second Tier: Sometimes a girl feels that she won't be loved by anybody and nobody will find her interesting and worthwhile. Then she discovers that her sexuality seems to arouse a lot of attention, especially from young men–and maybe from some young women. Well, that's an important discovery, now she has some way of getting people to notice her, think about her, want her–and even if all they want is to use her, even if that's their only interest, still, they want her for a while, for now–and that's a lot better than not to be wanted at all.

Third Tier: Underneath all that stuff, you think of yourself as damaged, worthless, and unlovable. No one would really want you, your own mother threw you out. And that thought hurts so much that you try to turn it away by saying: I'm so cute, so sexy, that everybody wants me. And you keep yourself busy with these sexy games and activities–and then you don't have to face that inner part of you that yearns to be mothered, that feels so worthless, and that tells you that nobody could really want you.

In that connection, there is a special dimension of this that takes the form of wanting to be pregnant. Many very troubled and deprived teenage girls assert this wish in an insistent way from very early on indeed. This is always scandalizing to staff members: My god, they say, this child can't take care of herself and lurches through life from one self-engendered catastrophe to another. What will she do with an infant, what damage will she cause to another life, and what damage will she herself sustain if she carries through with this plan? Within the therapeutic setting, this wish for pregnancy is usually expressed in the form of a declaration: I think I'm pregnant! With the inevitable ensuing flurry of blood and urine tests, and investigations to determine who her sexual partner was and how come it happened, where was the staff?–when all that has been gone through and it turns out–as it usually does–that she is not pregnant but wishes she were and declares her determination to achieve that goal–what then does the staff say?

First Tier: You seem real disappointed that you are not pregnant. That sounds like a mighty powerful yearning.

Second Tier: You talk about it as though being pregnant would solve all your problems. You would have a baby to love only you, and you could love the baby all you wanted to and it would all be a wonderful feeling all the time.

Third Tier: For a long time, you have had a terrible hunger to be mothered and cared for and loved, just for yourself alone. The hunger is there because you never got that–or enough of that–when you were an infant. So now you want to ease that pain and satisfy that hunger by having a baby of your own that you can make it up to–you can give to that baby what you never got and what you never stopped longing for–it seems like an answer to all the loneliness and emptiness and the unloved feelings in your life.

In brief, the effort is to make the youngsters turn inward, to urge them to seek the solution to their difficulties by self-understanding, to help them by knitting together the past with the present, to make their motives and their behavior meaningful and coherent. This kind of work has to come at them from everywhere; this is the strength of milieu. They are thus englobed in therapy–and so serious are their conditions, that often enough, nothing less will do.

This then is one way that psychoanalytc principles can be translated into milieu usage. Training staff to work in this way would in time go far to professionalize child care work and lend additional credence to the assertion that the contribution of the staff is critical to the resolution of these grievous conditions. Setting up such training seems a game worth the candle.

REFERENCES

Gunderson, J. G. (1989). Personality Disorders, Introduction. In: Karasu, T.B. *Treatment of Psychiatric Disorders: A Task Force Report of the American Psychiatric Association. Volume 3.* Washington, D.C.: The American Psychiatric Association.

Kernberg, O. (1984) *Severe prsonality disorders: Psychotherapeutic strategies.* New Haven: Yale University Press.

Kohut, H. (1971). *The analysis of the self: A systematic approach to the psychotherapeutic treatment of narcissistic character disorders.* New York: International Universities Press.

Marohn, R., Dalle-Molle, D., McCarter, E., and Linn, D. (1980). *Juvenile delinquents: Psychodynamic assessment and hospital treatment.* New York/Brunner/Mazel.

Masterson, J.F. (1972). *Treatment of the borderline adolescent: A developmental approach.* New York: Wiley.

Millon, T. (1981). *Disorders of personality: DSM-III: Axis II.* New York: John Wiley & Sons.

Ornstein, A. (1981). Self-pathology in childhood: Developmental and clinical considerations. In: K. Robson (Ed.), *The psychiatric clinics of North America: Development and pathology of the self (Volume 4, pp. 435–453).* Philadelphia: Saunders.

Rinsley, D.B. (1980). Diagnosis and treatment of borderline and narcissistic children and adolescents. Bulletin of the Menninger Clinic, 44, 147-170.

Residential College as Milieu: Person and Environment in the Transition to Young Adulthood

Bertram J. Cohler
Susan E. Taber[1]

The place of social context in determination of wish and action continues as a focus of study within the social sciences. Perspectives from the study of lives over time have suggested that the important factor in the relationship between person and context is the implicit or subjective interpretation of environment experienced in terms of personal goals and concerns. Kurt Lewin's (1935,1947) concept of "life-space" and Murray's (1938) conception of personal need and both subjective and objective environmental force or press expresses this conception of experienced place as significant for personal adjustment and morale. Bettelheim's (1943, 1960, 1980a) discussion of the power of the concentration camp to change personality has provided further evidence of the significance of this experienced environment or milieu as a factor determining the experience of self and others.

Relying upon his reflexive understanding (Kohut, 1959; Schafer, 1969; Gardner, 1983), regarding his own and others' experiences in the concentration camps, Bettelheim used this understanding in the construction of a milieu for troubled young people which would express this power of the experienced environment as a factor contributing to therapeutic change in a positive manner. Bettelheim's (1950, 1955, 1973) pioneering study of therapeutic intervention at the University of Chicago's Sonia Shankman Orthogenic School stressed the subjective significance of both space (architecture) and time (structure of the day, including transition times) in facilitating enhanced personal control over a world experienced as overwhelming.

The concept of milieu is founded on the psychoanalytic study of wish or intent and feeling or sentiment, extended through the work of Bettelheim (1943, 1950, 1955, 1960), Bettelheim and Sylvester (1948, 1949), and Redl and Wineman (1950, 1951) to residential treatment designed for children and adolescents. From the consideration of the meanings of designs on gift-wrapping paper on birthday presents to the design of stairwells and hallways as transition spaces, Bettelheim's concern with milieu or the meaning of the environment for mental health, contributed not only to the psychoanalytic treatment of troubled children and adolescents, but also to a theory of person and environment, fostering morale and enhanced personal integration.

The therapeutic milieu is designed to reduce the press upon children and adolescents which had propelled them into actions unacceptable to family and community, reflecting intense personal distress. A similar model has been developed on an empirical basis by Stern (1970) and by Stem, Stein, and Bloom (1956), showing the impact of environment upon personality and action. More generally, environments may be viewed in terms of the extent to which they promote enhanced personal development and foster increased sense of personal integrity or congruence which is so essential for effective performance. While the concept of milieu has most often been regarded in terms of its significance for psychotherapeutic intervention, it is possible to extrapolate from principles underlying the concept of milieu to other group living situations concerned with planned interventions. The college residence hall represents one such planned intervention setting in which the whole environment provides potential for fostering optimal development.

It should be emphasized at the outset that this perspective does not imply that the college should undertake the unreasonable burden of being "psychotherapist." However, recognition of the mental health implications of going to school, more generally, may foster the role of school and college in realizing its potential (Cohler, 1989; Cohler and Galatzer-Levy, 1992). The mental health significance of education is implicit in such diverse aspects of the college experience as the student's relationship with both fellow students and with faculty. For example, students reenact experiences over a life-time with those viewed as "being in charge" within both classroom and residence hall (Cohler and Galatzer-Levy, 1992). Recognition of the significance of these enactments may assist both residence hall staff and instructors in understanding particular student difficulties and in working with these difficulties without any explicit discussion of these problems having occurred.

PSYCHOLOGICAL MILIEU
AND PERSONAL DEVELOPMENT AND CHANGE

The concept of milieu is important in understanding personal development and change within those settings such as schools and colleges which are the focus of such deliberate interventions as education or psychotherapy (Cohler, 1989; Cohler and Galatzer-Levy, 1991). The residential liberal arts college is one environment designed to promote personal and intellectual development (Ekstein and Motto, 1969; Jones, 1968; Sanford, 1962, 1966). Many of the forces assumed to foster the transition from adolescence to young adulthood are highlighted in the American residential college, which is unique in its concern with an integrated view of such personal and intellectual development.

Relying upon the concept of milieu as portrayed both by Bettelheim and his colleagues (Bettelheim and Sylvester, 1948, 1949) and by Redl and Wineman (1950, 1955), it is possible to view the residential college as a milieu and to gain increased understanding of the significance of the residential college in fostering emergence of personal and intellectual maturity in the lives of young adults (Heath, 1968). This article discusses the particular significance of the undergraduate residence hall or "college house" in the transition from adolescence to young adulthood,[2] extending Bettelheim's concept of milieu to the study of the college residence hall.

The college residence hall is one kind of milieu, or total personal and physical environment, functioning to provide opportunities and constraints upon personal and intellectual development to maturity. The central problem confronted both by the college residence and by residential treatment concerns the anonymity and compliance with external constraints which is imposed by group living within an institution.[3] The problem in each instance is that institutional living may foster conformity and reduce sense of personal control over the environment. The problem with institutional life, whether residential treatment or residential college, is the preservation of a sense of personal autonomy and control in a setting demanding conformity to group pressure (Bettleheim, 1960) and conformity to decisions made on the basis of the best interests of the setting rather than the concerns of those living within it. Recognition and response to implicit concerns and interests of individuals within the group setting make it possible for the total environment to work toward promoting maturity.

THE CONCEPT OF MILIEU

Bettelheim's concept of "milieu" was founded on his study of the concentration camp and the impact of such an extreme situation upon both intent and action. The concentration camp represents the "ideal type" (Weber, 1904-05) of a milieu explicitly designed to foster extreme behavior. Bettelheim's classic (1943, 1960) report on mass behavior in extreme situations elucidates the manner in which even the most minute details of the physical and interpersonal surround were designed to reduce personal autonomy and to create an experience of helplessness and despair. Bettelheim realized that if environments could be so structured that they exercised such destructive impact upon personality, then it could be possible to construct a milieu which had the opposite effect, that is, fostering enhanced sense of personal autonomy and integration.

The concept of milieu includes both those persons who live within it, and the architectural spaces in which they live, including the symbolic attributes of the physical space and the subjective meanings attributed to persons living within this environment. Person and setting act in concert in order to foster enhanced personal development, including both experience of increased integrity and realization of plans and intentions within the context of satisfying relationships with others.

Recognizing the complex nature of the relationship between institutional climate and personal development and, particularly, perceived constraint or press exerted by the surround upon wish, sentiment, and action, George Stern and his colleagues have developed a means for classifying college environments. Although Barker and Wright's (1951) classic study of the typical day of a boy in a midwestern community, and similar studies reported by Gump, Schoggen and Redl (1963) and Schoggen (1963), had shown that environments could be portrayed in terms of their significance for participants, Stern's work represents the most complete and detailed effort to portray the relationship between personal significance and institutional context.[4] Stern's (1970) discussion extends this perspective across a variety of colleges and provides additional support for the assumption of a "best-fit" between student expectations and college opportunities and constraints. Some students prefer the anonymity and autonomy of life-style provided by a large state university campus, and may even prefer the less personal educational climate of the large lecture hall, while other students seek the greater sense of community and personal recognition possible in a small liberal arts college.[5]

COLLEGE MILIEU AND THE TRANSITION FROM ADOLESCENCE TO YOUNG ADULTHOOD

The application of the model of the therapeutic milieu pioneered by Aichorn, Bettelheim and Sylvester, and Redl and Wineman, extends from the classroom to work place and other institutional settings; one particular setting in which the milieu concept becomes particularly informative is the residential college dormitory. Concern with the issue of milieu may be most significant at critical points in the transition across the course of life when the role of context becomes particularly important in fostering response to challenge to present adjustment.

The transition from high school to college mirrors the larger transition recognized in our society from adolescence to young adulthood. Even if not yet assuming the complex expectations of adults, young adults are expected to be able to realize the roles of work and marriage, and at least to anticipate the advent of parenthood. Historical and cross-cultural study suggests that recognition of a point in the course of life between attainment of biological maturity and assumption of adult roles is unique to our own time within bourgeois Western society (Demos, 1986, Demos and Demos, 1969). Recognition of a time between childhood and adulthood in which boys and girls attained maturity and the knowledge to participate as members of the adult social order was first possible with the publication of G. Stanley Hall's (1902) two-volume work on Adolescence. Across the succeeding century there has been much study of the adolescent epoch from both medical and social science perspectives. However, it is only in our own time that a second epoch, that of youth, has been recognized as preceding the phase of settled adulthood (Cohler and Boxer, 1984).

First portrayed by Erikson (1958, 1961, 1968) and Keniston (1960, 1963, 1968) as youth, the developmental tasks unique to this epoch include consolidation of identity and self-definition of career or vocation, and realization of enhanced capacity for intimacy. Arnett and Taber (submitted) have enlarged upon this concept of youth as "emerging adulthood," referring to the period defined by a partial completion of the role transitions of adulthood including completion of formal education, the taking on of full-time employment, marriage and parenthood. Increased time spent preparing for vocation, lack of support within contemporary society for the transition into the work-force, particularly within urban American society, and social changes making assumption of non-traditional roles and alternative lifestyles possible, have all contributed to increased range of personal choice. Increased number of lifestyle choices have emerged at the same time that more traditional means, such as the apprenticeship for getting started in the labor force, have largely disappeared in contemporary urban society.

Social changes unique to our own time have led to the recognition of youth as a time characterized by a distinctive crisis or challenge to continued development to psychosocial maturity (Havighurst, 1952). Young adults are expected to make commitments to career and intimacy, and to assume responsibilities within the larger society which require a preparatory period which is made possible either through military service and/or college.[6] Elder (1987b) has shown the significance of military service for the lives of an earlier cohort of men attaining adolescence after the Great Depression. Having phased out the draft for military service, post-secondary education is the only institutionalized means presently available for trying-out roles and life-styles prior to having to make a commitment to a particular pathway into settled adulthood.[7]

Negotiation of the relationship with parents is somewhat less constrained and difficult among students living apart from parents while at college. Further, as in so many aspects of the transition from adolescence to young adulthood, the presence of others experiencing the same developmental challenges provides an opportunity to reflect upon available options and to learn from peers struggling with similar issues (Goethals and Klos, 1970). Residential life, in which beginning and more advanced students live together may play an important role in socializing younger students into college culture and may provide the informal guidance which is unique to the peer group. Nevertheless, there are continuing problems of continuity and change which are pronounced within the college culture.

Many young people are able to make the transition from high school to college with relatively few problems. However, at least to some extent, this transition to college reflects aspects of response to an extreme environment (Sanford, 1968). Although offering opportunities for the newly found freedom of adult life, the university in turn requires autonomous performance with little supervision. The often anonymous and impersonal nature of the university as an institution experienced along with continuing concerns regarding the welfare of parents, often many thousand miles away (too many upper middle-class parents announce plans to get a divorce only as their offspring are getting ready to go off to college), and the disruption, loss, and change characteristic of the move to a new environment (Marris, 1974), all pose a challenge for even the best adjusted student. Among more intellectually able but psychologically fragile students, the transition to college becomes an overwhelming experience leading to psychological symptoms much in the manner portrayed by Bettelheim and Sylvester (1948, 1949) and Bettelheim (1950, 1955). Residential life may play an important part in ameliorating these feelings of being overwhelmed and may facilitate the adjustment from home to college.

While much of the focus of college is upon intellectual preparation, the college experience includes more than the classroom. Indeed, study suggests that many of the most important aspects of a student's experience in college take place outside the classroom (Katz, 1968a), particularly in the residence hall or dormitory. While there has been at least some study of the college classroom, there has been much less study of the contributions to liberal arts education of the college residence. Findings from systematic study of higher education (Newcomb, 1943; Newcomb, Koenig, Flacks, and Warwick 1967; Feldman and Newcomb, 1969; Katz and Associates, 1968; Heath, 1968) suggest that residential life makes important contributions in student growth to maturity and that more detailed consideration of the place of residence life within the context of the college as a whole would both enhance the educational mission and provide increased understanding of the impact of context upon personality development and change across these formative years of youth.

The paucity of study of residential life is due largely to the uncertain status of residential life within the college, which is as old as the concept of a "college." From the first founding of European universities, the definition of education has been restricted largely to classroom and laboratory; too often residential life has been regarded as "auxiliary" in terms both of budget and staffing (Cowley, 1934).[8] However, it is difficult for the college or university to assume that the residence hall is only "auxiliary" when considered in the light of findings showing that out of classroom activities account for the greatest intellectual and personal development across the college years (Sanford, 1962, 1966).

THE RESIDENTIAL COLLEGE AND THE UNIVERSITY

Discussion of the college residence as pivotal in the transition from adolescence into young adulthood, assisting young people to resolve salient developmental issues involves questions both regarding the mission of post-secondary education and also objective and experienced constraints and opportunities provided for young men and women attending college. The place of residential living within the college or university has been the subject of continuing discussion since the founding of the first universities in the middle ages. Even assuming responsibility for providing accommodations for students, there has been a continuing question regarding the relationship of residential life to the intellectual mission of the university: while the prevailing view of the college house emphasizes the opportunity provided for attainment of personal and intellectual maturity, means for attaining this goal most often have not been specified.

The Place of the Residential College Within the University

Cowley (1934) has provided a definitive portrayal of the emergence of the American residential college based largely on the English Oxbridge (Oxford and Cambridge) model. Cowley notes that the idea of a college residence was not initially linked with the emergence of the university on the Continent but that problems in student self-governance soon led the university to assume responsibility for residential life. However, as early as the Enlightenment, tensions developed between both instructional and budgetary resources for classroom and residence which soon led universities to abandon the concept of the residential college. The French Revolution continued across the Nineteenth Century as a reminder of the dangers inherent in a student culture fostered by residential life as a potential source of additional agitation.[9]

Since many of the American colonial leaders had been graduates of the Oxbridge tradition, the first American colleges, Harvard and Yale and William and Mary emulated the Oxbridge tradition of university sponsored residential housing. The need for college sponsored housing was further dictated by the paucity of local accommodations, the age of these colonial college students (often three to four years younger when beginning college than present day first-year students). Students often travelled long distances to attend college; it was obviously essential that the college should provide housing for these students.

Later, across the Nineteenth century, with the emergence of the public land-grant university in the Midwest, the model of the residential college had little acceptance.[10] It is likely that the American university would have moved in the direction of the Continental university with accommodations totally separate from the college or

university were it not for two other distinctively American develop-
ments in post-secondary education. Recognition that a democratic
society required collegiate education for both men and women led
to emergence of the "woman's college" in New England across the
last half of the Nineteenth century (particularly Mount Holyoke,
Vassar and Wellesley.) Obviously, the college would have to
construct housing since Victorian manners dictated that young
women could not be left unchaperoned in the community.

The second influence was the emergence of the private university
outside of the Northeast, particularly the University of Chicago.
Influenced by Yale's long-standing commitment to the concept of a
residential college, when William Rainey Harper founded the University of Chicago on a swamp at the time of the Columbian Ex-
position, he planned dormitories as an integral part of the Quadrangles.[11] From the outset, Chicago's influence in higher education
was significant, and Harper's commitment to undergraduate housing spurred other colleges to reconsider the significance of residential life within the larger university.

The place of residential life within the larger university remains a
continuing conflict within American higher education.[12] From the
outset, it was recognized that creation of a residential program
necessarily involved supervision of student life. Indeed, when students first asked the university to manage the crowded quarters
which students had established at Bologna and Paris, financial over-
sight was soon followed by supervision of student conduct within
the residence hall. What was unique about the Oxbridge experience
was the effort to integrate instruction and residential life. While the
colonial American replication of the Oxbridge model at Harvard
and Yale included the concept of the residence hall, it did *not*
include this integration of instruction and residential living which
was also central to the Oxbridge model (Cowley, 1934; Rudolph,
1962/1990; Jencks and Riesman, 1963). While faculty living in the
Oxbridge College houses developed close personal relationships
with students, fostering student scholarship through frequent individual tutorials emphasizing critique of written work, the Puritan
ethos determined that housing supervisors be more concerned with
discipline and moral life than with education.

First American colleges established the norm continuing in most liberal arts colleges to the present time: instruction takes place in the classroom while the dormitory is viewed as a place for relaxation and recreation supervised by staff concerned with maintenance of order. From the colonial time to the present day, American college faculty have had little contact with the dormitory system; a student-faculty reception is a major social event often marked by uncomfortable efforts on both sides to make "smalltalk." The lives of students and of faculty are so separate that conversation beyond classroom topics becomes strained and difficult to sustain.[13]

Sustained efforts at integrating education with dormitory living emerged quite late in the history of American higher education and have been confined largely to Harvard and Yale whose integrated program of residence and education has only been realized within the past half century. While it is often assumed that this college-house system was long the model of elite private higher education, emergence of the college-house as both residence and place of instruction by a faculty formally attached to the college residence is largely the outcome of concerns expressed both by Harvard's President Lowell and Yale's President Hadley that increasing emphasis upon graduate education across the last-half of the Nineteenth century had led the university to neglect its traditional commitment to undergraduate studies.[14]

The Harvard-Yale house system fostered construction of elegant college houses providing inviting and comfortable accommodations, with a distinguished senior faculty member or Master, assisted by other residential and non-residential faculty and graduate-student tutors, providing both classes and individual student tutorials. Relatively little disciplinary responsibility was expected within an atmosphere of liberal learning in which students were assumed to be mature. Just as in the older Oxbridge tradition, disciplinary issues were left to a staff of porters responsible for the maintenance of the house.

With the exception of Oxford-Cambridge in England and the Harvard-Yale college house tradition in the United States, the predominate model of the undergraduate residence has been one of a "hotel" rather than an integrated "college house system" approach. Particularly when state universities have been located in small communities, large scale dormitory construction in the postwar era has led to residential towers often housing more than a thousand students. Across recent decades, staffing patterns have shifted to the wide-spread use of other students as "monitors" or "assistants." These towers are staffed almost entirely by other students whose responsibility is defined largely as maintaining order and insuring an atmosphere conducive to studying and sleeping (Moffat, 1989).

Particularly when liberal arts colleges are a part of a complex research university, residential life becomes an important element of undergraduate education, complementing and extending the classroom, providing students with an opportunity to discuss ideas in an atmosphere less competitive and constrained than the lecture hall. The Harvard-Yale house system model has shown that faculty presence in the residence system through tutorial classes, shared discussion at meals, and discussion sections of large courses complete and enhance the classroom experience, fostering student integration of the diverse elements which comprise post-secondary education. Indeed, if the most significant aspects of a student's experience in college take place outside the classroom, then it is particularly important to extend instruction beyond the classroom into those areas of students' lives which are most significant for them.

Fostering Development to Maturity Within the Residential College

The liberal arts college is designed as a time of challenge leading to personal and intellectual ferment encouraging students to reconsider prevailing assumptions. Studies of higher education (Heath, 1968) suggest that this goal is attained; students report that courses in English, Psychology, and Philosophy have had particular impact upon their personal and intellectual development. Too often, this curriculum is not offered in a measured way, or with sufficient support. Students often feel unsupported and alone as they attempt to make sense of contradictory perspectives which may pose serious personal and intellectual challenge (Cohler, 1992). Sanford (1966) observes that the experience of being challenged in core assumptions may be personally disruptive for students.

While some critics (Bloom, 1987) complain that college is insufficiently intellectually stimulating, Sanford's observations suggest that encounter with new ideas, in the absence of support for such inquiry, may be overwhelming for intellectually able but psychologically fragile students. To date, other than Heath's (1968) study, there has been little systematic inquiry regarding the impact of curriculum upon students, and even less consideration of the role of residence staff in assisting students to manage the impact of the subjective aspects of the curriculum (Cohler, 1989; Cohler and Galatzer-Levy, 1992).[15] It is important to distinguish between the objective or explicit and the subjective or implicit meanings of the curriculum (Dewey, 1930; Katz and Sanford, 1962; Jones, 1967; Katz and Henry, 1988; Cohler, 1989). The objective curriculum refers to the subject matter taught, and the presumed direct impact of this teaching upon student competencies,[16] whereas the subjective refers to the psychological experience of having one's assumptions challenged.

Concern with issues of personal achievement, with being judged by both faculty and peers, and problems with self-esteem in which disappointment follows success when few attainments ever match personal aspirations, all represent issues which must be confronted within both classroom and residence. Obviously, more psychologically resilient persons are able to deal with threats to self-esteem and competition with greater success, sometimes even enjoying the very competitiveness involved in scholarship. Particularly within the natural sciences, where grading is according to the "curve," and where some students must inevitably get average or lower grades, issues of competition and self-worth may be particularly intense. Once again, institutional and personal characteristics are interrelated; some educational institutions are particularly concerned with the human side of learning and advancement of knowledge, while others foster competition and enhance a sense of personal inadequacy.

Struggle with these issues is not limited to the classroom. Indeed, many of these issues first emerge within the context of the dormitory. Particularly in an intense intellectual climate, student experience of lowered self-esteem as a consequence of struggling with work far more difficult than in high school leads to a continuing sense of inadequacy. Recognition of this problem on the part of residence staff is an important aspect in the contribution of residential living to the student's capacity to perform in the classroom (Kohut, 1984). As one student observed to his resident head, after "unloading" a series of doubts regarding academic competence, it was helpful to have someone who was willing to listen. The experience of being listened to is among the least studied but most important aspects of psychological intervention (Kohut, 1977, 1982, 1984). The experience of being listened to fosters enhanced selfcongruence and is requisite for the willingness to undertake more sustained study of personal distress.

However, listening is more difficult than may appear.[17] Attuned listening supposes the capacity in the listener to bear own tensions, maintaining an empathic stance (Kohut, 1959; Schafer, 1959; Gardner, 1983) and to be reflexively aware of wishes and fears reciprocally stimulated by student problems (Flarsheim, 1975). Among residence staff, many of whom may be dealing with similar issues in their own undergraduate or graduate studies, discussions concerning self-esteem and academic competence may resonate with their own concerns. Assuming the role of resident staff assumes a certain degree of self awareness, including recognizing and understanding their own wishes and feelings as a part of a process of continuing self-inquiry (Gardner, 1983). This awareness on the part of residence staff is essential in maintaining the capacity for empathic understanding of students.

Staffing for the College Residence. While there has been extensive discussion of staffing for the college residence (De Custer and Mable, 1974), little discussion has been devoted to the psychological significance of this residence staff position for both staff and students with whom they work. Generally, residence staff consists of well intentioned and interested doctoral students or undergraduates. Indeed, as Greenleaf (1974) has noted, colleges are increasingly turning to undergraduates as primary staff members because of the expense involved in recruitment of more experienced and mature staff. This is unfortunate because, in the first place, student needs and expectations may be burdensome, particularly at times when student-staff also have exams to take and papers to write. In the second place, complex issues of competition often arise, particularly when third and fourth year students of the same age as student residence staff live in the same college house. One student-staff member noted the problems arising from being in the same classes as those for whom she was supposed to be responsible. Not only was there increased competition, but also the student staff member felt continually "on duty," performing in an exemplary manner in the classroom and the dormitory at the same time that students with whom she was working worried that her academic success would "raise the (grade) curve."

Development of social and intimate relationships between student staff and those whom they are supervising is an awkward issue. Student staff are expected to develop social relationships outside the house. However, with little free time it is difficult to realize this expectation. Too often, complex problems arise when student staff become close friends or intimately involved with students whom they are supposed to be supervising. The line between being open and becoming too seductively close is a difficult one for a student to realize and requires considerable maturity and self-awareness.

Clearly, long-standing historically and culturally determined reluctance of the university to become involved in the lives of students may contribute to a haphazard staffing system. However, there is also an enduring belief that the role of residence staff is to facilitate the student's own struggle to realize personal maturity while that of the faculty is to foster development of intellectual skills. Implementation of this goal is best attained through a low-key, informal role for housing staff (Commission on Professional Development, Council of Student Personnel Association, July, 1972). The assumption that "less is better" too often pervades efforts to intervene on behalf of a student's struggles to realize goals. Particularly where the sole residence staff consists of other undergraduate students in a residence of as many as a thousand students, staff expectations necessarily must be limited.

Finally, just as with faculty, students may idealize the resident head or the resident assistant in ways which it is difficult for them to accept. At least some faculty choose to avoid undergraduate teaching because undergraduates express admiration which faculty, uncertain of their own self-worth, find difficult to tolerate. Student admiration may make faculty acutely aware of their own feelings of not living up to their own ideals for themselves (Cohler, 1992; Cohler and Galatzer-Levy, 1992). These issues may become magnified in the residence hall lacking the classroom formality which is able to provide distance between student and staff. Expressions of admiration for the accomplishments of the residence staff may make staff members acutely aware of their own doubts regarding their own accomplishments, leading them to depreciate themselves in the eyes of their students. In the effort to maintain their own precarious self-esteem through idealization of housing staff, students may intrude in ways not always appropriate, asking residence staff questions which may be embarrassingly personal. Again, students may attempt to idealize their residence staff and seek to emulate the model provided by staff. There may even be requests to borrow clothes or other possessions in an effort to model themselves on these idealized residence staff.

Co-educational Residential Life. The shift in values which has taken place across the past decade has led to further problems in residential life. Reviewing a number of Carnegie Commission surveys of higher education, Levine (1980) has documented changes in student attitudes regarding life-styles over the course of the preceding two decades. Coeducational residence, a utopian dream only a few years previous (Rimmer, 1968), was an accepted reality by 1970. However, shared residence has posed problems as well as opportunities for both men and women. Two first-year men students recounted problems in learning to shave with a hand razor. Looking into the bathroom mirror, they saw two women students, who were waiting for a shower, giggling at them. These two young men found the experience mortifying!

Students are expected by their room-mates to find other places to study and sleep when their roommates are entertaining lovers. However, it may be difficult to find a friend willing to tolerate disruption of schedule in the midst of an assignment which is due the next day, and the makeshift living arrangements may make it difficult for both students to concentrate. Wishes stimulated by finding a roommate in bed with another student pose additional issues, particularly among students early in their college career. While it is sometimes assumed that a form of "incest taboo" exists within a college house, students within a college house may develop intense intimate relationships which sour after a period of time. Encountering former lovers on a daily basis may pose a tension for both the former couple and other members of the house.

Other more serious problems posed for students by co-residential living include realizing a sense of intimacy, regulation of sexual wishes, having to confront such alternative life-styles as gay consociates, and the shift from parental to self regulation of wishes which has been without parallel over the past century (Elson, 1986). As long as parietal rules governed the hours at which women were required to return to the college dormitory, and staff monitored visits to the dormitory of the other gender, there was both less opportunity and also lessened challenge of having to deal with issues of sexual intimacy. While, to some extent, a part of the inevitable crisis of the first collegiate year has always concerned monitoring the use of time, with parents no longer available to "nag" about homework, and, at least on the urban campus, increased opportunity for other social and personal experimentation, the new freedoms of the past decade have required increased student maturity and personal responsibility. For some time, recreational drugs have been much more available to college students than previously and, at least until the adoption of 21 as the legal drinking age across the nation, increased opportunity for drinking as well.

At the same time, as Katz (1974, 1987) has noted, co-residence also provides new opportunities for students to realize satisfactions from relationships. Living with another, sharing personal and sexual intimacies, provides increased opportunity for closeness, empathy, and the satisfaction obtained from a loving relationship during the college years. Many of the problems involved in fostering this capacity for intimacy are portrayed in Goethals and Klos' (1970) collection of student "first-person" accounts regarding relationships between college age men and women. These autobiographical accounts document the pathos as men and women struggle to realize satisfying intimacy and to deal with issues of sexual closeness in the context of rapid social change in expectations regarding intimacy in the college years.

As these first-person accounts show, co-educational residence has enabled both men and women to prepare themselves for the reality of adult life in which previous distinctions between the work of men and women has diminished. Students engage in working out issues between men and women which, a decade earlier, would have been expected among married couples. Opportunity for living together adds particular intensity to relationships, requiring both men and women to confront the meaning of intimacy. Further, while men in liberal arts colleges with large numbers of women, such as Sarah Lawrence or Vassar, have accepted the reality of women as intellectual equals, women face a greater struggle than men in realizing such acceptance at many co-educational private and land-grant institutions. Over time, co-residential living should lead men to become more comfortable with a view of self which includes doing tasks formerly assumed to be a part of the woman's world; women may gain increased courage undertaking careers previously assumed to be the province of men (The Brown Project, 1980).

Komarovsky's (1976, 1985) longitudinal studies of co-residential living among undergraduate men and women at Columbia University provides some support for this claim that co-residential education has had a continuing positive impact on the manner in which young men and women understand self and others. At the same time, at least among men, there was a continuing sense of strain attempting to adjust to new ways of relating to women, some sense of uncertainty in intellectual discussions, and enhanced concern regarding adequacy in sexual relations. Often, an early serious relationship between a man and a woman was a response to continuing conflict with parents. These relationships reflected efforts to create for oneself a missing sense of family.

A decade later, studying Barnard undergraduate women, Komarovsky (1985) reports that many of these earlier concerns had disappeared. Among the women in her study, perception of the relation among men and women was more equalitarian than a decade earlier. The Womens' movement appears to have had additional impact upon both attitudes of women and men in an elite college. Over the course of the four college years, these women increased their commitment to career, rather than marriage and family, following college graduation. However, more traditional women, non-careerist in orientation, were less certain of their own occupational goals and more critical of the Women's movement for its intolerance of a life-style focused on marriage and family. Women electing careers were more often from families in which their own mothers were dissatisfied homemakers. Komarovsky also reports a marked shift among women at this elite college towards more explicitly acknowledged interest in sexual activity, although only in the context of a caring relationship. Women still seem more concerned than men with a close connection between sexuality and interpersonal intimacy.

Residential Life and the Transition into and Out of College. Heath (1968) and Perry (1968) have reported that the freshman is often both shocked by college and challenged and threatened by the diversity of background and life-style encountered in the elite liberal-arts college. The transition from high school to college may be as significant a role transition as that of marriage or first full-time job. Levin (1967) notes the particular problems posed for students living in residential colleges, living away from home and learning to relate to roommates. Particularly among students living away from home for the first time, "homesickness" may be embarrassing. Some students may become envious of younger brothers and sisters still able to live at home, or worried about problems such as parental illness or marital problems. If problems develop at home after the offspring has left for college, there may be increased feelings of responsibility either for having "caused" these problems or for not being home to be of help. One first year young woman announced tearfully to her resident head that her absence from the family was the cause of her teenage brother's suicide attempt.

Coelho, Hamburg, and Murphey (1963) note that the transition to college means encountering new subject matter in unfamiliar areas of study, increased demands for intellectual performance, need to master new skills, often with the additional time pressure of examinations, increased requirement for self-regulation of time such as that for homework, and commitment to extracurricular activities in ways more consistent with the adult world than that of high school. Studying a group of particularly competent students during the senior year of high school, after selecting colleges ranging from the local state university to elite New England colleges and, again, after starting college, these authors report that successful transition to college was associated with enhanced self-esteem. Students coping more successfully with this transition selected colleges more appropriate in terms of their ability. Once arriving on campus, these more competent students relied upon academic skills already acquired in high school, constructing a story of college interests based on continuity with high school accomplishments. These students were able to develop reasonable expectations regarding academic success, based on interests, difficulty of courses selected and extracurricular interests; they did not need to make perfect grades in every course.

Students more successful in making the transition from high school to college were also able both to concentrate in a new environment and to fit their own work with the interests of instructors with whom they were studying, focusing on intermediate rather than long-range concerns, and to seek advice and support, both from other competent first-year students and more advanced students and from faculty. These students sought to model themselves on particularly admired instructors, using this admiration as an additional source of strength in their own struggle to learn. More competent students were able to find instructors to admire who supplied what they believed to be missing attributes of self. One student, disappointed in his relationship with a father whom he saw as not very effective, was able to select an instructor as a role model who had realized considerable success in his field and who enjoyed helping students attain similar success. Finally, these more competent students also showed a playful attitude towards the process of learning and were able to maintain reasonable expectations regarding what they could achieve. They could modulate disappointments in their own success, through emphasizing areas in which they were academically strong, and through increased participation in those extra-curricular activities such as athletics or music which supplied them with an enhanced sense of accomplishment. The residence hall presents an important opportunity for finding experienced students and staff to adopt as role models.

The transition to college may be seen by some students as an extreme situation. Particularly among intellectually gifted but more troubled young men and women, the response to the developmental challenge posed by the transition from adolescence to youth, marked by beginning college, may be experienced as beyond their capacity for mastery. The press of this challenge may lead to construction of a false self leading to a sense of personal depletion and despair which may lead to desperate efforts to maintain some feeling of being alive through sensation-seeking experiences such as through substance abuse and dangerous and provocative behavior. Feeling unable to live up to their own ideals and expectations, and feeling too personally depleted to use the college experience, these students turn to any stimulating experience which will help them feel alive.

Findings regarding the senior year of college, including transition from college to career, pose a greater paradox and provide less consistent findings. Studying women in an elite women's college, and reflecting more generally on the college experience, Sanford (1966) suggests that college seniors experience more marked disruption in sense of self than students at any other point across the college years. Confronted with the necessity of making a transition from college to the "real world," fourth year students go through prolonged periods of questioning personal goals and career choices.

At least to some extent, Sanford's portrayal conflicts with Heath's (1968) study of personality development across the college years: by their senior year, Haverford students showed enhanced sense of self and increased concern regarding the welfare of others. While an earlier study of women in traditional women's colleges (Freedman, 1956) suggested that women had little difficulty during the senior year, since they expected marriage and parenthood as the next step in the transition to adulthood, this may be less the case at the present time. Over the past two decades, with changing attitudes towards women and career or vocation, women are confronting the same problems as men have traditionally faced. They, too, increasingly rely upon vocation as confirmation of their integrity and self-worth, seek fulfilling work in their first job after college, and are subject to the same work strains as their masculine counterparts. Evidence of this work strain is beginning to appear in studies of stress and adult health, including increased cigarette use among educated women (Cohler and Galatzer-Levy, 1992).

RESIDENTIAL COLLEGE AS MILIEU:
PERSPECTIVES FROM THE CHICAGO EXPERIENCE

This discussion of the concept of milieu relevant to college residential life is based on residential life in an urban midwestern university with a distinctive educational philosophy. The University of Chicago was founded in 1892 by William Rainey Harper, using funds provided by oil baron John D. Rockefeller. As Cowley (1934) has noted, a part of Harper's "experiment" was the explicit inclusion of college dormitories in his initial plan for the Quadrangles. Distinctive of this university was its immediate rise to international stature as a research university through the immediate purchase of an internationally renowned faculty. Although most often celebrated for the first American research university, based on his experiences at Yale, where questions regarding the place of the residential college within the larger university were already being discussed, Harper also maintained distinctive views regarding the importance of undergraduate education, including the significance of a residential college within the larger university. Hutchins' assumption to the University's presidency in 1929 led to the most significant revolution in the liberal arts curriculum of our own time. Together with Harper's initial vision, Hutchins' educational reforms highlighted the mission of the liberal arts college within the larger research university (Levine, 1950/1992).

Harper planned dormitories as an integral part of the Quadrangles. Indeed, Chicago has been unusually fortunate in being able to provide both residential housing for all students, including unusual variation ranging from the more supervised life of the residence hall to independent student apartments (as is common at most liberal arts colleges, first year students are required to live in the College residence halls). However, virtually from the time of its founding, as in so many American research universities which also include a liberal arts college, Chicago has experienced continuing tension between the goals of a scholarly community and the instructional needs of an undergraduate college. On the other hand, particularly since the presidency of Robert Maynard Hutchins from 1929-1951, Chicago has been known for its distinctive general education program which was largely staffed by European teacher-scholars in exile, generally without departmental appointments in their home disciplines.

The seriousness of purpose which is a self-conscious element of Chicago's educational climate, and the combination of the University's continuing commitment to an extensive and rigorous general education program, together with the excellence of its academic programs and research facilities, continues to attract a group of unusually talented and serious college students. One of the few institutions of higher learning in the world in which an undergraduate is able to knock on the office door of a Nobel prize winner, Chicago's undergraduates would rather discuss classical texts or take on additional work in a research laboratory than attend a dance or go on a ski trip. In ways characteristic of many American universities, Chicago has too often assumed that undergraduate instruction interferes with programs of research and writing; there has been little explicit concern within disciplinary programs with undergraduate instruction or with the concerns of these students as young adults struggling with both intellectual and personal concerns.

Recognizing the particular nature of the expectations which students place upon themselves, and which lead them to be attracted to a college such as Chicago, an intellectual perspective founded on concern with the significance of the concept of milieu for personal and intellectual development is important in understanding the contribution of the college residence in the personal and intellectual development of those students who select this particularly intense college. Bettelheim (1950, 1955, 1960) and Bettelheim and Sylvester (1948, 1949) have maintained that much of what is known as personal distress or psychopathology could be understood as response to an extreme situation.

The two-thirds of students living in College housing are supervised by a staff of resident heads who are generally advanced doctoral students, university professional staff or College student advisors, and residence assistants, who are advanced undergraduate and beginning graduate students. Recognizing that these undergraduate students represent an unusually motivated group of students who subject themselves to immense psychological pressure in an effort to live up to their own ideals, residential life at Chicago fulfills a particularly important mission within the larger university. If Chicago is often experienced by students as a psychologically extreme environment, the residential college system provides a milieu in which enhanced academic attainment and growth to personal and intellectual maturity may be facilitated.

The implications of this unique college environment for student personal development has been documented by Stern, Stein, and Bloom (1956) who have documented the "Press" (Murray and Associates, 1938) or experienced tensions concerning personal and intellectual development which exists at Chicago. These problems include the extent to which students are expected to structure their own educational objectives, and the extent to which these objectives are realized, the variety of subject matter in which students are expected to acquire academic competence, the extraordinary degree to which even beginning undergraduates are expected to relate to faculty at the highest level of scholarly sophistication, the relatively minor role played in student life by traditional extracurricular college activities such as athletics and fraternity life (Chicago students continue to regard the graduate research library as the student social center), reliance upon encounter with primary source texts and contemporary research literature rather than textbooks as the foundation of learning, and the extent to which students continually judge each other, and are evaluated by their instructors, on the basis of articulate participation in class discussions and particular sophistication in written work. Indeed, it is assumed that even first-year undergraduate students are capable of significant scholarly attainment.

Recognizing the very high level of intellectual distinction which students expect of themselves at Chicago, within a university in which all members of the community, from first year student to senior faculty, continually demand the utmost in scholarly achievement, students at Chicago encounter an intellectual climate seldom found in the American university. The problems posed by this distinctive college environment for student adjustment have been documented by Stern, Stein, and Bloom (1956), Yufit (1957), Isaacs (1957), and Isaacs and Haggard (1959). Particular problems emerge for those students who are somewhat less dedicated to intellectual pursuits, and less self-initiated, in their approach to their college education. Additional problems arise among those students more generally concerned with ideas than with people, who find it difficult to relate to others and, often, who experience problems maintaining self-esteem and living up to unusually high goals regarding scholarly attainments.

Students with a more traditional intellectual, political, and social orientation find this challenging environment demanding creative thought to be particularly difficult. Yufit (1957) additionally reports on the high degree of intellectual and personal isolation which characterizes the personality of college students struggling to attain important intellectual goals in an educational climate which demands unusual personal and intellectual maturity.[18] Cohler (1989, 1992) and Cohler and Galatzer-Levy (1992) have further documented the costs in terms of adjustment demanded by an unusually rigorous intellectual climate which taxes capacity for personal integration. Among students with already weakened self-esteem, an intellectual climate as taxing as Chicago can foster disturbance of personal integration manifested either by depletion depression (Kohut, 1977), or by construction of a false self (Winnicott, 1960) in which there is superficial effort to comply with the expectations of a world felt as overwhelming, leading to the experience of personal disintegration reflected in intense personal distress including episodes of major psychiatric illness.

Among liberal arts colleges, where students have continuing contact with faculty in small classes, and where the campus is sufficiently small that students can know each other, residential life may play a less important educational role (Heath, 1977). The necessity for this integration of classroom and residence hall is particularly important when considering the developmental tasks of late adolescence and young adulthood. Central among these tasks are realization of goals for work or vocation, enhanced capacity for intimacy, and realization of a new relationship with parents and other family members as members of a family of adulthood.

The incoming student at Chicago is in a particularly vulnerable position, seeking to realize young adulthood yet confronted with diversity in life-style, enhanced academic pressures, and concerns regarding personal adequacy which may be compounded by problems at home prior to leaving for college. A majority of students in many college houses come from stem or reconstituted families. The financial strain inherent in attending an expensive, elite liberal-arts college poses challenges for virtually all families planning for their college education (more than two-thirds of Chicago students work, generally in excess of nine hours a week, in order to help pay for their education–the largest proportion of scholarship and working students among the elite liberal arts colleges). Where custody or other conflicts between divorced parents further interfere in providing for education, the student's own college career becomes jeopardized.

Many of the issues posed by problems at home and in the college classroom become the province of college residence staff. Often, with young adults involved in similar struggles with their parents, they are both in an unusually fortunate position of listening to these problems, but also personally challenged by these issues. The so-called dormitory "bull-session" is an important element of residence as milieu. In the first place, these sessions share with the marginal or life-space interview (Redl and Wineman, 1950, 1951) the immediacy of time which fosters intensity of both event and conversation about the event. In the second place, students may be able to say things to each other, and to be of help to each other in ways not possible to realize when staff talk with students one-on-one. However, in order to maximize this opportunity, there must be a place where students come together for those discussions which observational and systematic study has both highlighted as among the most important of the factors leading to personality change and intellectual development in college.

It is important that the living room be as home-like and non-institutional as possible. Among the most important aspects of Bettelheim's discussion of milieu was his concern that institutional life interferes in the development of personal autonomy. It is particularly important that the residence milieu on the college campus be as home-like and personal as possible. An environment fostering personal autonomy rather than the anonymity of an institution facilitates comfort and conversation. Provision of books about the city, guides to area restaurants, and train and bus schedules provides students with enhanced sense of connection with their new found surroundings and provides encouragement for students to think about exploring the neighborhood and the near-by city. Posters referring to college and area history additionally foster a sense of pride and connection with college and city in a manner similar to the decals of their college logos which many students purchase and place on their family car.

Staff availability, particularly just prior to dinner or after dinner, and in the late evening, also provides encouragement for students to drop-by and talk about their concerns. Particularly when students return to the residence hall from the library, finding a receptive house living room, with other students present and students and staff with whom to talk, provides a welcome alternative to return to a house in which doors are all shut and there is no one around with whom to 'talk (a view which is consistent with Bettelheim's (1950) discussion of transition times within the milieu). The very presence of concerned and attentive staff available for listening facilitates student opportunities to rework and integrate the experiences of the preceding day. Late-evening study breaks provide a particularly important opportunity for the "bull-session" which all studies of personality and intellectual development across the college years note as particularly significant for enhanced personal and intellectual development. These are but a few of the ways in which the concept of milieu therapy may be applied in a non-intrusive manner to fostering change within the residential college.

Where possible, use of the resident head living room as a place for house members to gather may facilitate these conversations. As students wander in and out, particularly in the evening, a range of issues comes up for discussion which would not be possible in any other context. Ranging from anxiety in dating and forming relationships, to such problems at home as a brother or sister moving into the absent student's room and using the prized stereo, an unfortunate classroom experience, or larger political and social concerns, these marginal or "life-space" interviews (Redl and Wineman, 1951) are central in group life and uniquely provide both understanding and support for students.

Attainment of a sense of personal integrity is a primary developmental task of the college years (Erikson, 1958, 1963). Many of the issues pertaining to both vocational and sexual identity are most dramatically posed within the residence. Much of the concern with vocational identity is focused around the issue of the college concentration program or "major." The issue of switching concentration areas is closely tied to the issue of vocational identity. An issue of particular concern is that of the "pre-medical" student whose own identity has been closely allied with the healing arts. Often, these students have been pressured by their family into electing careers in medicine for personal or financial reasons. Coming to college, these students begin to question their previous decision, and to explore options in other fields. One student discovered a fascination with Renaissance history and, after a period of self-doubt, decided upon graduate study rather than medical school. The students's parents were distressed with this decision and pressured him to reconsider his goals. Several evening sessions were devoted to discussion among students regarding their own reasons for selecting a concentration program and to problems with parents whose own anxiety on behalf of their offspring at a time of national economic recession had led them to become particularly careerist. With the support of his peers and the residence staff, the student was able to maintain his commitment to doctoral studies focused on the history of medicine in the Renaissance with the possibility of later completing medical education together with graduate studies.

Issues of sexual identity are among the most complex and difficult of all issues confronted within the residence milieu. Problems of co-educational living have been further compounded by recent concerns regarding "political correctness" and focus on the issue of stigma and stereotyping among erotic minorities. At the same time, this renewed concern with the plight of those students possibly subject to stigma has made it possible for students to discuss issues of sexuality and sexual identity in ways not previously possible. One student who had attended an experimental public high school was particularly distressed upon coming back to his room and finding his roommate engaged in sexual intimacy with another man student. Further, his roommate had just come "out" and received calls from other homosexual students at all hours. Even though this student had been aware and acceptant of a homosexual life-style from his urban high school experiences, this more immediate encounter posed problems in dealing with his own sexual identity and orientation and disrupted his concentration upon his work. Referral to the University's Student Resources and Counseling Center was of great value in assisting this student to deal with these conflicts.

Unusually good communication between the house system at Chicago and the Student Resources and Counseling Center facilitated the process of finding a therapist with whom to discuss these issues. This incident also shows the importance of attaining greater sensitivity to the personal meaning posed for students by the equally important effort to increase sensitivity to issues of stigma and discrimination based on sexual preference. It is important to be aware of the psychological conflict posed for students by the imposition of required programs heightening student sensitivity to issues of gender and ethnicity. Too often, residence staff, responsible both for residence life education and for dealing with student tensions regarding these issues, are expected both to implement programs presumed to foster enhanced student sensitivity without sufficient recognition of complex issues involved for students and staff alike in discussing these issues. Particularly among younger residence staff, their own personal struggles with such issues as sexual identity and orientation and intimacy poses problems in dealing with these issues among students.

CONCLUSION

The concept of the therapeutic milieu was initially framed as a means of understanding the totality of environmental forces leading to personality change. Initially the consequence of Bettelheim's observations regarding the disastrous impact of the concentration camp (Bettelheim and Sylvester (1948, 1949), Bettelheim (1950, 1955, 1960), and Redl and Wineman (1950, 1951) led to this concept of residential treatment within the milieu, recognizing the totality of environmental forces fostering positive personality change. Another milieu, the college residence has been shown to have a directed impact upon the lives of college students posing both problems and opportunities in group life, especially the problem of institutional conformity which may interfere with personal development.

The college residence has occupied a marginal place in higher education. Residential life and classroom have been kept separate for much of the history of higher education. From the time of the first universities in the middle ages, there has been continuing tension between formal instruction and student life outside the classroom. This tension is due in part to the distinction first made in the Enlightenment between the realm of the rational-intellectual and the personal or other than rational aspects of learning (Weber, 1904-05; Jones, 1968; Ekstein and Motto, 1969; Cohler, 1989; Cohler and Galatzer-Levy, 1992), as well as problems assumed to be posed both by having a group of young people living together and the attendant issues of "emotional contagion" (Redl and Wineman, 1951) which may lead to disruptive behavior, and also the personal demands made on faculty by working with students in an informal basis outside of the classroom. Indeed, with the exception of Oxbridge in England and Harvard and Yale in the United States, and a very small number of experimental colleges such as Deep Springs College in the California desert, students go one direction and faculty go another direction after class. All too often, failure to integrate classroom and residence deprives students of the possibility for meaningful education and deprives faculty of the opportunity to impact intellectual and personal development among students.

A truly residential college challenges students and faculty alike, and makes additional demands upon college resources. Faculty may be threatened by student efforts to idealize them since such idealizations may run counter to the personal concerns of faculty somewhat uncertain regarding their own personal and intellectual attainments. Just as residence staff, faculty encountering student problems and concerns may find it difficult to listen to these problems in ways which are not personally threatening. While issues of the personal significance of student concerns may be assumed to be a part of the "job description" of residence staff, they are not usually considered in faculty recruitment based largely on intellectual attainment.

Finally, increased recognition of the significance of the college residence as a force of both personal and intellectual development across the college years poses demands upon university administrators for both additional funds in order to rehabilitate the physical plant and increased effort to recruit personally reflexive and mature staff for the college residence. These staff require additional support from such other college resources as student counseling and student health services. In order to realize the promise implicit in residential life, student residence facilities must be more closely integrated within the context of the larger institution than at the present time. More effective integration of classroom and curriculum with residential life promises to foster student personal and intellectual development and to reduce feelings of student estrangement from both classroom and instructor commonly reported within the contemporary college and university. Faculty as well as students may gain from this additional interchange; faculty have a unique opportunity for understanding the manner in which students make use of what they learn in the classroom, and are challenged to provide for ever more effective teaching.

It is time to reconsider the traditional tension between classroom and residence and to more effectively integrate the college residence within the milieu of the college as a whole. This more effective integration promises increased value of the undergraduate education and increased effectiveness of the college in realizing its mission of fostering personal and intellectual development across the college years. If the most significant learning takes place outside the classroom, as study of higher education has suggested, then it is time to take advantage of the milieu as a whole in order to foster student development. Some guidelines for this more effective integration of classroom and residence have been provided through the study of the therapeutic milieu.

Bettelheim's (1950, 1955, 1973) discussion of issues in the more effective integration of classroom and dormitory in a children's residential center is relevant in this discussion. For example, problems of both transition space and transition time, and of the difficulties faced by children as they move from dormitory to classroom and back is also an issue for students at college. The transition from dormitory to classroom, with different expectations and different demands becomes evident, for example, in problems faced by students considering whether to skip class in favor of some other activity.

A psychoanalytically informed approach to the study of the relationship between classroom and residence, relationships among young people and staff, and to selection and staff education, adds a distinctive perspective in settings as diverse as residential treatment and the residential college. Too often, it is assumed that such a perspective requires unusual staff education. In fact, this approach merely highlights the importance of understanding implicit as well as explicit significance in communication, and in developing the capacity for empathic listening based on a modicum of self-reflection and inquiry. A psychoanalytic perspective is important in understanding the phenomena of the milieu, and in guiding efforts at most effective intervention.

Particularly within the setting of the residential college, the best intervention may be attentive listening to student concerns fostering student efforts to realize solutions for problems which they confront. Students comment that the presence of a good listener facilitates their own enhanced self-understanding and effort to solve problems which they face with instructors and school work, roommates and friends, and home and family. Continuing staff self-reflection or inquiry provides a good guide regarding the most helpful or useful intervention appropriate within what Redl and Wineman (1950, 1951) have portrayed in their report on milieu intervention as the marginal or life-space interview. Within the residential college is the need to attend to implicit as well as explicit communication, to foster the sense of personal effectiveness and integrity, and to maximize opportunities for enhanced personal and intellectual maturity.

NOTES

1. The authors are resident heads within the house system of The University of Chicago. Largely a result of the inspiration of Edward Turkington, presently Deputy Dean of Students, the Chicago college-house system has emerged uniquely in American higher education with a system of adult resident staff concerned primarily with fostering students' personal and intellectual development. The authors are grateful to Dean Turkington for having created a house system implicitly recognizing concepts of milieu and appreciating the significance of the collegiate experience in fostering the student's intellectual and personal development. Obviously, our perspective on the college residence as a milieu represents only our own views regarding the place of the college residence in undergraduate education.

2. The cultural symbolism involved in the use of the term "house" used to describe the college residence hall is significant for the present discussion, as is the Latin term "Alma Mater," used to refer to the college itself. At least within

American culture, concepts of home and family have been extended to college itself; the college is the mother and the college residence the house which replaces the family home. Meals are taken together "family style" and students live in the kind of personal relationships which are likely to characterize family life. The irony, of course, is that relatively few students have realized the family life portrayed as ideal within this culture. Nearly three-quarters of the students living in our college houses came from disorganized or reconstituted families, typically those in which parents had divorced and each remarried other divorced parents with children, or those in which the father had deserted the family and, too often, even refused to pay college tuition bills.

3. The problem of conformity is particularly significant within the college residence hall. While many liberal arts colleges require one year of residence in the dormitory, in most colleges students are free to seek other accommodations after the first year. While some students return to live at home, most students choose either to remain in the residence hall, to live in independent off-campus housing or, in schools with a strong "Greek" system, to live in a fraternity or sorority house. Reviewing findings from the study of personality and growth to psychological maturity across the college years in an elite liberal arts college (Stanford), Lozoff (1968) has reported that those students electing to remain in the dormitory system tended to be more conformist and passive in their orientation to others than students electing to live off-campus or in fraternities. At the same time, students electing to continue to live in the college houses were more likely to undertake graduate study in the arts and sciences in preparation for a scholarly career while students electing to join fraternities were most likely headed for careers in law, business and medicine. Students electing fraternities were most likely to have leadership potential and to enjoy taking initiative in student activities. Those electing off-campus life tended most often to be nonconformist, rebellious and found it difficult to live in any group situation. Lozoff's findings show again the fit between personality and social context in which persons find those living situations which are most congenial and supportive of their own personality. These findings also show the problems posed by dormitory living for students electing dormitory residence. The problem is that the institutional conformity imposed by this group living is all too consistent with their own personal conformity and may not foster enhanced sense of personal vitality and spontaneity of the more mature and creative adult which these students also seek to become.

4. Studies in the tradition of ecological psychology founded by Barker and Wright (1951) make many of the same assumptions regarding the significance of the environment for adjustment as the milieu formulation of Bettelheim (1943, 1950, 1960) and Redl and Wineman (1950, 1951). Following Lewin's (1935, 1947) classical theory of social field forces acting upon persons, milieu and ecological perspectives assume that the life-space, as the psychologically significant environment, plays an important role in determining individual behavior (Gump, Schoggen, and Redl, 1963). Residential treatment and residential college life share in common concern with the life-space as a factor influencing both action and intent. Environments reflecting caring, respect for person, and the

importance of psychological vitality, autonomy and responsibility, lead to enhanced experience of personal integrity and to socially responsible actions.

5. Finally, although there has been little study of this issue, prospective students are quick to evaluate potential fellow-students upon a first visit to a campus, and are usually able to make an immediate decision regarding the suitability of a particular campus for their own college career. In terms of the present discussion, these applicants are quick to determine whether they will receive the support and affirmation which they seek within a particular educational environment.

6. While college was an option realized by only a small number of middle class men in prior generations, in our own time more than half of young adults seek education beyond high school. Post-secondary education is widely recognized as an essential element of preparation for careers in contemporary society, and as market for the selection of mates (Holland and Eisenhart, 1989).

7. Countries such as Israel still requiring the military or other national service typically interpose this service between high school and college. A period of national service provides an opportunity for exploration of adult roles prior to college. As a consequence, students are more mature when beginning college and are able to settle upon particular career decisions earlier in a post-secondary education which is less concerned with moral education than the American system with its stress on general education or core-curriculum.

8. This distinction between residential life and education parallels the distinction so often made in residential treatment between the "therapy hour" and the "other 23 hours." Too often, there is a problem in recognizing the milieu as a planned and directed intervention either in psychotherapy or in education.

9. Cowley (1934) suggests that England's relative isolation from the political and intellectual revolutions taking place on the Continent may have protected "Oxbridge" from those changes which marked the end of University sponsored housing on the continent (problems in providing sufficient accommodations in the small cities of Oxford and Cambridge may also have played a part in fostering the concept of a residential college). Adelman notes that, in addition, Church control of the two major English universities both provided sufficient funds for academic and residential programs and also pressure to retain this structure more generally within English intellectual life. With the advent of the red-brick universities in the Nineteenth century, first efforts to provide only education without accompanying residence become problematic since, again, the cities in which these new universities were located did not have sufficient housing for large numbers of students seeking admission. Further, although it had been assumed that most students would be commuting from home, these universities soon attracted students from across the country. Charitable efforts to provide housing soon yielded to a national scheme for the provision of residence as integral to the planning of the university although not always accompanied by the faculty tutorial system of Oxbridge (Adelman, 1969).

10. Cowley (1934) and Rudolph (1962, 1990) both note the hostility towards a residential college model expressed by Henry Phillip Tappan, the influential mid-Nineteenth Century president of the University of Michigan who had studied at a

German research university and was impressed with the system of student residence outside the university. Indeed, Cowley (1934) quotes the observations of Henry Frieze, a colleague of Tappan at Michigan, that Tappan believed student dormitories would lead to disorderly conduct and the need for constant supervision, and that the college dormitory was anti-democratic.

Tappan's views were widely followed by other land-grant college administrators who were reluctant to commit scarce financial resources to construction of student housing. Many had been to Germany as graduate students, where the concept of the research university was already well established, and were familiar with the continental pattern of non-college sponsored housing. These faculty and administrators may have been all too familiar with problems at those few American universities undertaking residence life through the middle of the Nineteenth century. Adelman (1969) has described the problems of supervising college dormitories where food-riots and student rebellions had become so commonplace that, by the end of the Nineteenth century, " . . . the majority of dormitories were converted into classrooms or demolished if the state of disrepair had gone too far." Finally, the emergence of the American fraternity and sorority system during this same time may have taken up some of the need for residence while rapid urbanization made possible increased number and variety of available housing for students at such urban colleges as Columbia in New York.

Tappan's critique of the residential college, supported by anecdotal information regarding problems of social control at colleges providing residential living, encouraged a pattern at emerging state universities in which students lived at home and commuted to campus. Again, improvement in public transportation and the automobile made commuting an ever more practical approach for the public university. The practice of living at home and commuting to campus has become common at many public universities. Cowley (1934) notes that as recently as 1900, there were virtually no college sponsored residence halls at any of the state universities. This pattern may still be observed both at Michigan, which has very little residential housing beyond the East Quadrangle, and the University of California which, with the exception of the Santa Cruz campus, has very little university sponsored housing anywhere in what is the nation's largest higher educational system.

11. Cowley (1934) reports that more than half of the buildings in the first construction at Chicago were college dormitories.

12. The problem posed by focus on the possible contributions of residential life to the overall mission of the college is that it may make both financial and staffing demands which may be difficult for the college to realize. Precisely because the dormitory has most often been viewed as auxiliary to the larger educational mission, the dormitory system is expected to be self-supporting. Indeed, since the enlightenment, continental universities have been unwilling to allocate funds to residential living which might be spent on instruction. At least in part, this separation between the intellectual and the personal in education represents the unfortunate heritage of the "new science" of the enlightenment in which formal instruction is seen as distinctively different from time out of classroom (R. Jones, 1968;

Toulmin, 1989; Cohler and Galatzer-Levy, 1991). Recruitment and education for college residence staff is too often informal and consistent with an effort to maintain a low profile in the college budget and to make few demands on scarce instructional or budgetary resources. If the concept of the milieu is accepted, then all aspects of residential life must be considered from room furniture to meal planning. At a time when most institutions are attempting to reduce expenses by contracting out dining services and even reducing dormitory repairs, requests for additional funds for residential living are not likely to be well received! From the perspective of the larger objective of a college education, this distinction between formal and informal learning interferes in the realization of the very goals intrinsic to a liberal arts education in the contemporary American college.

13. "Sherry-hours" formerly provided opportunity for students to invite faculty to house receptions; these receptions have been curtailed over the past decade as a result of the demand that colleges comply with federally mandated legislation regarding the legal age for drinking alcohol. Anecdotal observation suggests that sherry or wine fostered an ease among both students and faculty which is not as easily provided by a punch bowl or a coffee hour!

14. Woodrow Wilson attempted a similar plan at Princeton but was defeated in the effort by alumni loyal to the eating club tradition.

15. Findings regarding the personal and intellectual impact of post-secondary education have seldom considered the different effects posed for students at different points in their academic careers, or across post-secondary institutions differing both in institutional culture and in impact upon students (Stern, 1963, 1970). Much of the study of growth to personal maturity has taken place at elite colleges in the Northeastern United States, and shows increasing student tolerance of personal differences across the four years of college (Jacob, 1957). This change is more a result of out-of-class student contact, particularly in the college residence, than deliberate efforts of classroom instruction (Coelho, Hamburg, and Murphey, 1963; Lehmann, 1963). Findings reported in studies of personal and intellectual change across the college years suggest that much of the total change in understanding of self and place in society takes place within the first year of college, particularly the first half of the first year of college. The primary source of this change may be due to factors other than the objective curriculum (Sanford, 1962; Katz and Associates, 1968; Heath, 1968).

16. Much of recent critique in higher education has focused on the objective curriculum. For example, Bloom (1987) and Chaney (1988) both decry the declining significance of the "great text," which is claimed to inspire virtue in students through example. A contrary position, but one based on similar assumptions, emphasizes the significance of teaching non-western texts, and those by women, presumably as a means of enhancing student tolerance through increased appreciation of the "other." There is little evidence that these texts have the direct impact upon students which has been assumed, although Heath's (1968) study does suggest that the humanities and social science curriculum may be a source of personality change. Systematic study does show that the most significant factor contributing to enhanced maturity in ethical and moral concerns, as in most other

elements leading to enhanced personal maturity among college students is the out-of-classroom contact which they have with other students.

There is even less understanding of the role of subjective than of the objective curriculum. While Freud (1913) noted the significant contribution which education played in psychological development, there has been little study of this issue (Cohler, 1972a, 1972b, 1989). It is believed that learning the curriculum is enhanced as a consequence of dedicated teaching by enthusiastic, informed faculty, relying upon the discussion method in small classes marked by a democratic process (Lewin, 1947; McKeachie, 1962).

17. A very large literature on the contribution of in-service education for student staff (Brown and Zunker, 1966; Powell, Plyler, Dickson, and McClellan, 1969) has noted the importance of fostering listening skills and enhanced self awareness among student staff.

18. Indeed, in the first author's social science general education class, when discussing Holland and Eisenhart's (1990) study of two Southern colleges, students found it difficult to relate to the text. Students across the 28 sections of this common year course echoed similar themes: our students do not come to college looking for a husband (women students) or in order to have fun. With more than two-thirds of students on full scholarship, this relatively impoverished but unusually serious and academically talented group of students seeks only to realize their own intellectual goals.

REFERENCES

Adelman, H. (1969). *The Beds of Academe: A study of the Relation of Student Residences and the University.* Toronto: Praxis Books/James Lewis and Samuel.

Aichorn, A. (1935). *Wayward Youth.* New York: The Viking Press.

Arnett, J., Taber, S. (1992). Adolescence terminable and interminable: When does adolescence end? Submitted, *Journal of Research on Adolescence.*

Barker, R. (Ed.) (1963). *The Stream of Behavior.* New York: Appleton-Century Crofts.

Barker, R., Wright, H. (1951). *One Boy's Day.* New York: Harper and Row.

Bettelheim, B. (1943). Individual and mass behavior in extreme situations, *Journal of Abnormal and Social Psychology*, 38, 417-452.

Bettelheim, B. (1950). *Love Is Not Enough.* New York: Free Press/Macmillan.

Bettelheim, B. (1955). *Truants from Life.* New York: Free Press/Macmillan.

Bettelheim, B. (1956/1980). Schizophrenia as a reaction to extreme situations. In. B. Bettelheim, *Surviving.* New York: Random House/Vintage Books, 112-124.

Bettelheim, B. (1960). *The Informed Heart.* New York: Free Press/Macmillan.

Bettelheim, B. (1961/1963). The problem of generations. In. E.H. Erikson (Ed.) *Youth: Change and Challenge.* New York: Basic Books, 64-92.

Bettelheim, B. (1973). *A Home for the Heart.* New York: Knopf.

Bettelheim, B. (1980a). German concentration camps. In. B. Bettelheim, *Surviving*. New York: Random House/Vintage Books, 38-47.

Bettelheim, B. (1980b). *Surviving*. New York: Random House/Vintage Books.

Bettelheim, B., Sylvester, E. (1948). A therapeutic milieu, *American Journal of Orthopsychiatry, 8,* 191-206.

Bettelheim, B., Sylvester, E. (1949). Milieu therapy: Indications and illustrations, *Psychoanalytic Review, 36,* 54-68.

Bloom, A. (1987). *The Closing of the American Mind.* New York: Simon and Schuster.

Brown,W., Zunker, V. (1966). Student counselor utilization at four-year institutions of higher learning, *Journal of College Student Personnel, 7,* 41-46.

Chaney, L. (1988). The future of great books. Speech delivered to students and faculty in Fundamentals Program at the University of Chicago, October 1988.

Coelho, G., Hamburg, D., Murphey, E. (1963). Coping strategies in a new learning environment: A study of American college freshmen, *Archives of General Psychiatry, 9,* 433-443.

Cohler, B. (1972a). Psychoanalysis, adaptation and education. I: Reality and its appraisal. *Psychological Reports, 30,* 695-718.

Cohler, B. (1972b). Psychoanalysis, adaptation and education. II: The development of thinking. *Psychological Reports, 30,* 719-740.

Cohler, B. (1989). Psychoanalysis and education: III. Motive, meaning and self. In K. Field, B. Cohler and G. Wool (Eds.). *Learning and Education: Psychoanalytic Perspectives.* New York: International Universities Press, 3-83.

Cohler, B. (1992). Why read Freud? Psychoanalysis, "Soc. 2," and the subjective curriculum. In. J. MacAloon (Ed.) *General Education in the Social Sciences: Centennial Reflection on the College of The University of Chicago.* Chicago: The University of Chicago Press, 225-245.

Cohler, B., Boxer, A. (1984). Middle adulthood: Settling into the World-Person, Time, Context. In D. Offer and M. Sabshin *Normality and the Life Cycle: A Critical Integration.* New York: Basic Books, 145-203.

Cohler, B., Galatzer-Levy, R. (1992). Psychoanalysis and the classroom: Intent and meaning in learning and teaching. In. N. Szajnberg (Ed.)(1992). *Educating the Emotions: Psychoanalysis in American Culture.* New York: Plenum Publications, 41-90.

Coleman, J., and Associates. (1974). *Youth: Transition to Adulthood.* Chicago: The University of Chicago Press (Report of the Panel on Youth of the President's Science Advisory Committee).

Cowley, W.H. (1934). The history of student residential housing, *School and Society, 40,* 705-712, 758-764.

Demos, J. (1986). The rise and fall of adolescence. In. J. Demos, *Past, Present, and Personal: The Family and the Life Course in American History.* New York: Oxford University Press, 92-113.

Demos, J., Demos, V. (1969). Adolescence in historical perspective, *Journal of Marriage and the Family, 31,* 632-638.

Dewey, J. (1938). *Experience and Education.* New York: Macmillan.

Ekstein, R., Motto, R. (1969). *From Learning to Love to Love of Learning*. New York: Bruner/Mazel.

Elder, G. (1987b). War mobilization and the life course: A cohort of World-War II veterans, *Sociological Focus, 2*, 449-472.

Elson, M. (1986). *Self Psychology in Clinical Social Work*. New York: Norton.

Erikson, E. H. (1958). *Young Man Luther: A Study in Psychoanalysis and History.* New York: Norton.

Erikson, E. H. (1961/1963). Youth: Fidelity and Diversity. In. E.H. Erikson (Ed.) *Youth: Change and Challenge*. New York: Basic Books, 1-23.

Erikson, E. (1968). *Identity, Youth and Crisis*. New York: Norton.

Feldman, K., Newcomb, T. (1969). *The Impact of College on Students*. Volume I: An Analysis of Four Decades of Research. San Francisco: Jossey-Bass.

Flarsheim, A. (1975). The therapist's collusion with the patient's wish for suicide. In. P. Giovacchini, A. Flarsheim, and B. Boyer (Eds.) *Tactics and Techniques in Psychoanalytic Therapy. Volume II: Countertransference.* New York: Jason Aronson, 155-194.

Freedman, N. (1956).The passage through college, *The Journal of Social Issues, 12*, 13-28 (Special Issue, Personality Development During the College Years, N. Sanford, Ed.).

Freedman, M. (1967). *The College Experience*. San Francisco: Jossey-Bass.

Freedman, M. (1987). *Social Change and Personality: Essays in Honor of Nevitt Sanford*. New York: Springer-Verlag.

Freud, S. (1913). The claims of psychoanalysis to scientific interest. *Standard Edition, 13*, 165-192. London: Hogarth Press, 1955.

Freud, A. (1927/1946). *The Psychoanalytic Treatment of Children*. London: Hogarth Press.

Gardner, M. R.(1983). *Self Inquiry*. Boston: Atlantic Little Brown.

Goethals, G., Klos, D. (1970). *Experiencing Youth: First-Person Accounts*. Boston: Little-Brown.

Greenleaf, E. (1974). The role of student staff members. In. D. DeCoster and P. Mable (Eds.) *Student Development and Education in College Residence Halls.* Washington, DC: American College Personnel Association, 181-194.

Gump, P. Schoogen, P., Redl, F. (1963). The behavior of the same child in different milieus. In. Barker, R. (Ed.) *The Stream of Behavior*. New York: Appleton-Century Crofts, 169-202.

Hall, G. S. (1902). *Adolescence* (Two Volumes). Boston: Houghton-Mifflin.

Havighurst, R. (1952). *Developmental Tasks and Education*. New York: McKay.

Heath, D. (1968). *Growing Up in College*. San Francisco: Jossey-Bass.

Holland, D., Eisenhart, M. (1990). *Educated in Romance: Women, Achievement. and College Culture*. Chicago: University of Chicago Press.

Isaacs, K. (1957). Relatability: A proposed construct and an approach to its validation, Unpublished doctoral dissertation, The University of Chicago.

Isaacs, K., Haggard, E. (1959). Some methods used in the study of affect in psychotherapy, In. L. Gottshalk and A. Auerbach (Eds.) *Methods of Research in Psychotherapy*. New York: Appleton Century Crofts, 226-240.

Jacob, P. (1957). Social change and student values. *Educational Record, 41*, 338-342.

Jencks, C., Riesman, D..(1962). Patterns of residential education: A case study of Harvard. In. N. Sanford (Ed.) *The American College: A Psychological and Social Interpretation of the Higher Learning.* New York: John Wiley and Sons, 731-773.

Jones, J. (1974). Minority student concerns and cross-cultural relationships. In D. DeCoster and P. Mable (Eds.) *Student Development and Education in College Residence Halls.* Washington, D.C.: American College Personnel and Guidance Association, 117-134.

Jones, R. (1968). *Fantasy and Feeling in Education.* New York: New York Univrsity Press.

Katz, J. (1968a). *No Time for Youth: Growth and Constraint in College Students.* San Francisco: Jossey-Bass.

Katz, J. (1968b). Four years of growth, conflict and compliance. In. Katz, J., and Associates. *No Time For Youth: Growth and Constraint in College Students.* San Francisco: Jossey-Bass, 3-73.

Katz, J. (1974). Coeducational living: Effects upon male-female relationships. In. D. DeCoster and P. Mable (Eds.) *Student Development and Education in College Residence Halls.* Washington, DC: American College Personnel Association, 105-116.

Katz, J. (1987). Changed sexual behavior and new definitions of gender roles on the college campus. In Freedman, M. (Ed.) *Social Change and Personality: Essays in Honor of Nevitt Sanford.* New York: Springer-Verlag, 116-139.

Katz, J., Henry, M. (1988). *Turning Professors into Teachers: A New Approach to Faculty Development and Student Learning.* New York: American Council on Education: Macmillan.

Katz, J., Sanford, N. (1962). The cirriculum in the perspective of the theory of personality development. In N. Sanford (Ed.) *The American College: A Psychological and Social Interpretation of the Higher Learning.* New York: John Wiley and Sons, 418-444.

Keniston, K. (1960/1965). *The Uncommitted: Alienated Youth in American Society.* New York: Dell Books.

Keniston, K. (1963). Inburn: An American Ishmael. In. R. W. White (Ed.) *The Study of Lives: Essays in Honor of Henry A. Murray.* New York: Atherton-Aldine, 43-71.

Keniston, K. (1968). *Young Radicals.* New York: Harcourt, Brace, World.

King, S. (1973). *Five Lives at Harvard: Personality Change During College.* Cambridge, MA: Harvard University Press.

Kohut, H. (1959). Introspection, empathy, and psychoanalysis: An examination of the relationship between mode of observation and theory. *Journal of the American Psychoanalytic Association, 7,* 459-483.

Kohut, H. (1977). *Restoration of the Self.* New York: International Universities Press.

Kohut, H. (1982). Introspection, empathy and the semi-circle of mental health. *International Journal of Psycho-Analysis, 59*, 395-407.

Komarovsky, M. (1976). *Dilemmas of Masculinity: A Study of College Youth.* New York: Norton.

Komarovsky, M. (1985). *Women in College: Shaping New Feminine Identities.* New York: Basic Books.

Lehmann, I. (1963). Changes in critical thinking, attitudes, and values from freshmen to senior years. *Journal of Educational Psychology, 54*, 305-315.

Levin, S. (1967). Some group observations on reactions to separations from home in first-year college students, *Journal of the American Academy of Child Psychiatry, 6*, 644-654.

Levine, A. (1980). *When Dreams and Heroes Died: A Portrait of Today's College Student.* Jossey-Bass (Carnegie Council Report on Policy Studies in Higher Education).

Levine, D. (1950/1992). (Ed.) *The Idea and Practice of General Education: An Account of the College of the University of Chicago By Present and Former Members of the Faculty.* Chicago: The University of Chicago Press.

Lewin, K. (1935). *Dynamic Theory of Personality.* New York: McGraw-Hill.

Lewin, K. (1947). *Field Theory in Social Science.* New York: Harper and Row.

Lozoff, M. (1968). Residential groups and individual development. In. Katz, J., and Associates. *No Time For Youth: Growth and Constraint in College Students.* San Francisco: Jossey-Bass, 239-254.

McKeachie, W. (1962). Process and technique. In N. Sanford (Ed.) *The American College: A Psychological and Social Interpretation of the Higher Learning.* New York: John Wiley and Sons, 312-364.

Marris. P. (1974). *Loss and Change.* London: Routledge & Kegan Paul.

Moffat, M. (1989). *Coming of Age in New Jersey: College and American Culture.* New Brunswick, NJ: Rutgers University Press.

Murray, H.A. and Associates (1938). *Explorations in Personality.* New York: Oxford University Press.

Newcomb, T. (1943). *Personality and Social Change.* New York: Dryden Press.

Newcomb, T., Koenig, K., Flacks, R., Warwick, D. (1967). *Persistence and Change: Bennington College and Its Students After Twenty-Five Years.* New York: John Wiley and Sons.

Perry, W.G. (1968/1970). *Forms of Intellectual and Ethical Development in the College Years: A Scheme.* New York: Holt, Rinehart and Winston.

Powell, J., Plyler, S., Dickson, B., McClellan, S. (1969). The Personnel Assistant in College Residence Halls. Boston: Houghton-Mifflin.

Redl, F., Wineman, D. (1950). *Children Who Hate: The Disorganization and Breakdown of Behavior Controls.* New York: Free Press/Macmillan.

Redl, F., Wineman, D. (1951). *Controls from Within: Techniques for the Treatment of the Aggressive Child.* New York: Free Press/Macmillan.

Rimmer, R. (1968). *The Harrad Experiment.* New York: Phantom Books.

Rudolph, F. (1962/1990). *The American College and University: A History.* Athens, GA: The University of Georgia Press.

Sanford, N. (1962). Developmental status of the entering freshman In. N. Sanford (Ed.) *The American College: A Psychological and Social Interpretation of the Higher Learning.* New York: John Wiley and Sons, 253-282.

Sanford, N. (1962). (Ed.) *The American College: A Psychological and Social Interpretation of the Higher Learning.* New York: John Wiley and Sons.

Sanford, N. (1966). *Self and Society: Social Change and Individual Development.* New York: Atherton-Aldine.

Schafer, R. (1959). Generative empathy in the treatment situation. *Psychoanalytic Quarterly, 28,* 342-373.

Schoggen, P. (1963). Environmental forces in the everyday lives of children. Barker, R. (Ed.) *The Stream of Behavior.* New York: Appleton-Century Crofts, 42-68.

Stern, G. (1963). Characteristics of the intellectual climate in college environments, *Harvard Educational Review, 33,* 5-41.

Stern, G. (1970). *People in Context: Measuring Person-Environment Congruence in Education and Industry.* New York: John Wiley.

Stern, G., Stein, M., Bloom, B. (1956). *Methods in Personality Assessment.* New York: Free Press/Macmillan.

Toulmin, S. (1989). *Cosmopolis.* New York: Free Press/Macmillan.

Weber, M. (1904-1905). *The Protestant Ethic and the Spirit of Capitalism,* trans. T. Parsons. New York: Scribners, 1958.

Winnicott, D.W. (1960a/1965). Ego distortion in terms of the true and false self. In. D.W. Winnicott, *The Maturational Processes and the Facilitating Environment.* New York: International Universities Press, 140-152.

Yufit, R. (1957). Intimacy and isolation: Some behavioral and dynamic correlates, Unpublished doctoral dissertation, The University of Chicago.